For: ELISE

So you will know us better —

Enjoy and stay

Warm Regards,

5/14/91
X

... our apologies

The names, places and dates in this book are accurate to the very best of our knowledge. There may be some people who find that we have misspelled their names or misrepresented their titles, and for this we are truly sorry. If you send us a correction we will include it in the next printing.

In some cases we have taken serious exception to the behavior, treatment or attitude of various members of the medical world which we encountered during the management of Michele's illness. We wish to remind you that we in no way intend to convey, in this work, a blanket indictment of the medical field.

Without the dedicated and talented people who gave us their aid, their time, their skills and their love, we would not have Michele with us now. There are, however, certain medical practitioners whom we believe need to stop and examine the way they do business with real people, and make a major career adjustment. For guidance, a few of them are mentioned in this book.

That is why we say several times in this work: if you are not getting straight answers from your medical care giver, get up, walk out the door and find someone else — NOW.

We hope that you enjoy Michele's story and share it with others

— it was written for you!

Against The Odds

The True Story of Michele,
A Cancer Survivor

This work was written & experienced by

Patrick Nolan, her father
Patricia A. Nolan, RN, her mother
&
Michele K. Nolan, herself

First Edition
1995

Alchemy Publishing Company
"we turn words into gold"

2557 E. Sound View Drive
Langley, WA 98260-9740

Against The Odds

The True Story of Michele, A Cancer Survivor

Published by:
Alchemy Publishing Company
"we turn words into gold"

2557 E. Sound View Drive
Langley, WA 98260-9740
360-321-7705 • fax: 360-321-7980 • 800-831-3082

Copyright © 1995 by Michele Nolan

First Printing June 7, 1995

Printed in the United States of America

Cover Photo & Patsy & Patrick Photo: Teresa Vancosky
Back Cover & other B/W Photos: Patrick Nolan

Library of Congress Card Catalog Number: 95-76347

ISBN 1-887170-05-7 — $18.25 softcover

This work was lovingly edited by our good friend

Charlie Schwartz

Thanks, Chas. We could not possibly have completed this story without your wonderful suggestions, corrections, additions and thoughtful assistance.

Chapters

Dedications:

My efforts in this book are dedicated to:
Robert Filler, M.D., to Larry Page, M.D.,
to the staff of Childrens Hospital in Boston
and to a large black man who
worked in intensive care at Childrens
Hospital in Los Angeles twenty-five years ago.
I never knew his name,
but I will never, ever forget
his tender, gentle, loving touch
with my daughter.

Patrick Nolan

My contributions are dedicated to:
Dimetrius Traggis, M.D., Norman Jaffe, M.D.,
and to the lab technicians, nurses and staff at
The Jimmy Fund in Boston who held my hand,
wiped away my tears and helped me
through the terrible summer of 1969
...and for the next two years.

Patsy Nolan

I've decided to dedicate my part of this book
to my late grandmother, Lillian Whalen,
who knew all along that I would make it.
Thanks, Gram.

Michele Nolan

Throughout this work you will find some strong opinions about the care Michele was given, about the performance of selected medical professionals and other people who are mentioned by name or identified by location or by their job assignment.

These opinions and evaluations are solely those of the authors.

This work is written in three voices:
Patrick, Michele's father;
Patsy, Michele's mother
& later in the book,
Michele, herself.

Each time you see a double space between
paragraphs, the voice has changed.

Introduction:

We want you to know that this is not a story of suspense. It's a story of hopes and fears and togetherness — and a story of success. It's the intimate story of one family's battle with a deadly illness. It's the story of how our daughter, Michele Kathleen Nolan survived her battles with childhood cancer.

Michele is today a beautiful 30 year old young woman who has been completely free of the disease for over twenty-five years.

Michele wasn't a little girl who had her picture on the cover of People Magazine, having just been rescued from a well. She didn't appear on the evening news, searching desperately across the nation for a liver donor. She didn't attract the attention of the White House, a big sports celebrity or even a movie star.

Michele just lived through something that no one else has ever lived through.

When she was three years old, she developed a cancer of the kidney known as Wilm's Tumor. Eight months later, after two major surgeries to remove it, the cancer moved to her brain. As far as we have been able to discover, she is the only person to survive a Wilm's tumor of the brain. Or, as the doctors would say, an intercranial metastasis of Wilm's tumor.

Sometimes it's hard to believe that it's been twenty-five years since those terrible days and long nights when cancer invaded our sanity and scarred our very souls. Twenty-five years since the cold, white terror gripped our bones and made us tremble with fear and dread. Twenty-five years since Patsy and I held each other through the night, fearing that in the morning she would have slipped away...

...so briefly with us, now gone forever.

Of course, over the years we have told people about Michele's life and death struggle with cancer, but writing about it in all this detail, talking about each particular experience again, and remembering just how frightened we were, brings it all crashing back once more.

When you talk about it in general terms, it doesn't seem too tough. But when you take yourself back to a particular conversation with a doctor, or back to the night you had to tell your mom that her tiny granddaughter has cancer, or back to when we went to x-ray, recovery, ICU or any of those other places where death was lurking, it becomes clear, once again, that it was the most difficult experience of our lives.

We have decided to write this book because we want to reach out to parents who may one day find themselves trapped in that strange, medical world, alone on what amounts to an alien spaceship, with the life of their child hanging in the balance. We want to speak to the parents who are scared of everything, frightened of the doctors and the nurses, of the white and green world of medicine, and to the children and parents who can feel powerless in that cold, intimidating world.

We want to reach out to them and say, *"It's okay to question. It's okay to stomp your foot, pound on the table, yell, scream... do whatever you have to do, but get their attention, demand some straight answers and then make your own decisions. It's okay to take charge."*

There are lots of tears in this book. Some are tears of overwhelming and conflicting emotions and some are tears of terrible sadness, but there are also lots of tears of great joy.

...but, please, as you read this story, remember: through all the tears there was always hope. We never said that Michele's survival was in God's hands (although there were those who said that for us). We never said, whatever happens, happens for the best. We simply believed in our judgment to make the right decisions. We believed in each other and, most important, we believed in Michele, who you will discover as you read this book is one tough little cookie.

While this is the true story of a tiny little girl, now grown into a healthy, wonderful young lady, it's something more. It's the story of how a family, when faced with a series of terrible, frightening and seemingly overwhelming challenges, pulled together to conquer the terrible fear that comes with those frightening words — *your child has cancer.*

This is a story of hope, a story of tears, a story of courage and a story of luck. It's the story of how Michele and her parents helped one another get through a time of deadly seriousness.

Of course, it's also the story of the other children in the family, the grandparents and of the wonderful friends — some new, some old — who gathered around us during a time of black clouds and dark, frightening skies. It's also the story of how we discovered some very wonderful and very exceptional things about ourselves and about each other. It's even, in a very odd and wonderful way, a love story.

But this is mainly the story of Michele's successful battles with cancer.

Michele's story is being written now because, more than twenty years after she was first diagnosed as having cancer, Michele is finally ready to tell her story to others. She believes that it might help someone deal with a serious illness or give a little hope to those who might be feeling hopeless …especially a small, frightened child.

Michele's mother and father hope that the story of our experiences can bring some hope and encouragement to those who may today be where we were twenty odd years ago, standing there in a cold, white, brightly lighted hallway, feeling the marrow in our bones being sucked out as a doctor in a white lab coat calmly said to us, *I'm sorry, your child has cancer.*

So, if you, or someone in your family or someone you know — child or adult, is engaged in a battle with cancer or with some other life threatening illness, this book was written especially for you. We hope it helps, even if only just a little.

We're also writing this book because we would like to formally say "Thank You" to all those wonderful people who held our hands, gave us their love, fixed us a meal, handed us a cup of coffee, cleaned our house and shared our struggle.

Thank you, thank you all, for being there!

Before you read about her struggle,
let us assure you that today,
as we write this book,
"Michele is just fine, thank you!"

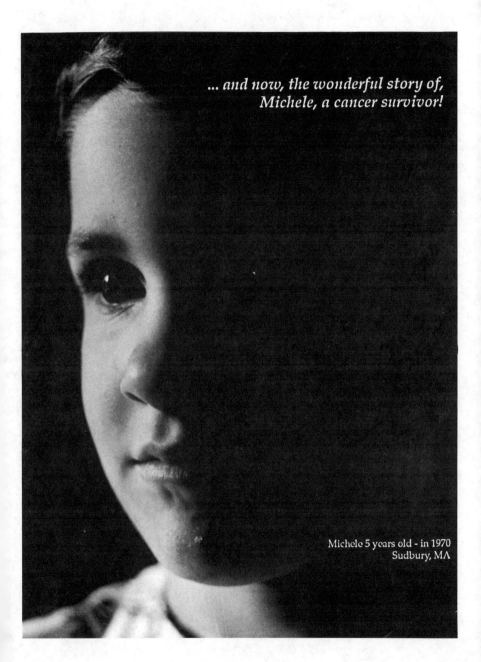

... and now, the wonderful story of, Michele, a cancer survivor!

Michele 5 years old - in 1970
Sudbury, MA

Our story begins in the fall of 1958,
seven years before Michele was born,
It begins the night Patricia Whalen, Registered Nurse,
meets Patrick Nolan, certified clown.

Chapter One

... and then, suddenly, she was with us!

While I've never regretted following my Aunt Pat into a career in nursing, I knew, early on, that I was not interested in emulating her spinsterhood. I was going to follow in my mother's footsteps and have a husband and a family. I have always loved nursing, but I didn't want my career to be my whole life. I wanted a husband and a family.

Back then, silly as it seems today, I sometimes felt that time might be running out on me. Here I was, an old maid in the making at the advanced age of twenty-three. As a number of my friends seemed to be pairing up in the first year or two after we graduated with our nursing licenses, I was anxious to find a partner.

I had had a couple of serious boyfriends, but I hadn't met anyone really special yet. Mom told me to be patient. Mom should know: she had waited until she was nearly thirty before she married my father. Even with what seemed like a very late start, they still found time to raise seven children. I wasn't ready to panic and marry the first guy who would have me, but I knew I was ready to start looking for "Mr. Right."

I was working as the Student Health Nurse at the St.Vincent Hospital School of Nursing in Los Angeles, when I accepted a blind date with a guy named, Patrick, one warm Saturday evening in October. Now this blind date didn't seem to hold much promise of being with "mister right,"but one never knows. And although I think blind dates are always a potential risk, this one seemed to be less threatening than most because I insisted that our friend, Don Williams and one of my roommates, Anita Tangaro, come along and make it a double date.

Don had been insisting for some time that Patrick and I meet. He had been telling me for months that Patrick was the perfect guy for me. Patrick was after all, according to Don, Catholic, rich and funny.

It turned out that Don was right for a few years about the Catholic part, but completely wrong about the rich part. He was, however, absolutely on the money about the funny part. Patrick has always been able to make me laugh, even on that first date, the only blind date Patrick would ever have with anybody.

When Patsy and I agreed to go on that first date, I was living 150 miles south of Los Angeles in the tiny desert town of Indio. I had returned to Indio after school in L.A. to join the family business with my Mom and Dad. At this particular time in my life, I wasn't the least bit anxious about getting married. At twenty-one I was having a wonderful time being a single adult — even if I was only just barely an adult.

Things changed on that fateful night in 1958, however; the night I met Patsy Whalen, RN. That night, I knew I was a goner. As soon as we met I knew that I would marry Patsy — if only she would have me. I had never met anyone who was that lovely, that gentle and that self confident. She had a natural beauty that began somewhere deep within her and flowed out through her eyes and her lips and her heart. I was, as the old Italians would have said, suddenly struck by "the thunderbolt."

Little did I know that the real thunderbolt in my life was waiting to strike me between the shoulder blades ten years down the road on a rainy November night, only a few miles away from where Patsy and I exchanged those shy greetings.

I never really asked Patsy to marry me. Probably for fear that she might come to her senses and say, no. But, asked or not, using good judgment or not, marry me she did, seven months after that first blind date.

On our wedding day, June 20, 1959, Patsy and I were seeing each other for only the twenty-second time in our lives.

There in the middle of a typical scorching summer day in the California desert, I stood at the altar, amused to be marrying the world's most beautiful — and surely one of the world's most nervous — brides. Later, my mother would say that Patsy looked like she had a small motor inside her as she knelt beside me.

After we were married, Patsy moved to Indio. We began our married life in a small two bedroom house, just across town from my folks' house and right next door to the family business — an eight lane bowling alley.

We spent the next few months getting a little better acquainted, getting used to living as a married couple and adjusting to a whole new lifestyle. I discovered that I really was completely crazy about my new bride. The thunderbolt had been right.

Before long, we decided to make a major change in our lives. What we proposed to do seemed to us to be very daring. At least it did in early 1960. We decided to pack up and leave Indio.

Our decision to move away began, I think, on the night our family bowling alley burned to the ground. That night was only a few weeks after our wedding. Not long after the fire, Patsy and I both knew that we had to leave Indio. Our new life together would have to be elsewhere.

The night the bowling alley burned down was a terrible night. It seemed like the entire town had been standing across the street from the fire with Patsy and my mom, watching our friendly little establishment go up in flames.

My Mom always thinks fondly of the atmosphere in our bowling alley when she sees the television program, "Cheers." The Indio Bowling Center, back there in the fifties, truly was a place where everybody knew your name.

The night of the fire Dad and I helped the volunteer fire department as they tried in vain to battle the incredible blaze. Unfortunately, stored in the back of the building were several twenty gallon cans of varnish and lacquer for surfacing the alleys. Those cans of volatile finish were exploding in the heat, further feeding the flames. Giant balls of fire would rise up out of the building as can after can of highly combustible wood varnish went off like napalm.

As the varnish and paint continued to feed the already desert-dry hardwood in the lanes, the fire was completely unstoppable. It was the most spectacular fire the town of Indio had ever seen. They say the flames reached up two hundred feet into the hot summer sky at their peak that night.

The interactions between Patsy and the rest of my family that night, and the fire, had a very special, almost profound effect on all of our lives. The tragedy brought Patsy crashing, full blast, into my family as a full fledged member. The fire acted as some strange sort of catalyst, helping melt the normal barriers which are, many times, to be found between a family and their newly acquired "in-law."

Although she had completely captured my dad's heart the very first night he met her, the fire demonstrated to my folks that Patsy had, with her heart, not just with words, cast her lot with us, forever.

While that night was certainly a night the town would not soon forget, it would be indelibly burned into the very soul of the Nolan family for all our days — and all our nights. Being a part of our family that tragic night — suffering with us the same sense of a deep personal loss — helped created a special bond between Patsy and my folks.

The night of the bowling alley fire was significant for another reason, too. It was the night that both of us, although we would not recognize it for many years, proved that we could count on each other to be there — no matter what cards might be dealt to us. That scorching night in 1959 was the night two people indeed became one. For the night the bowling alley burned down our marriage was, as some might say, truly tempered in fire.

While we may have lost a valuable family business that night, my folks gained a new daughter. But even more importantly, I gained a partner for life.

Even before the night of the fire, my dad had never referred to Patsy as his daughter-in-law. To him, Patsy was his daughter — period. The two of them had a very special, very precious love for each other, right from the beginning. But that night, both my Mom and Dad saw clearly that our loss was her loss, that our pain was her pain and that our fire was her fire.

While it's the goal of every young man to bring home to his folks a girl whom they will eventually love as much as he does, I had it so much better. Right from the beginning, my dad loved Patsy in a way that no one in our family, nor in Patsy's family for that matter, has ever clearly understood. To my dad, Patsy was his daughter, period. To her, he was, "Dad," period. She has never, in over thirty-five years, referred to him as her father-in-law. In fact, I don't think she has ever thought of him as anything but, Dad.

You must understand that Patsy loved her own father, Luke Whalen, as deeply as any father has ever been loved, but she and my dad had something between them which was very special and very precious.

While I was not a part of their special love for each other, I did enjoy watching it, for it was truly the loveliest gifts either one of them ever gave me.

A few months after the fire, Patrick's mom and dad took what insurance money was left after paying off the mortgage and the other bills and moved to Santa Barbara to run their newly acquired business, a neighborhood liquor store.

Patrick was working at the local radio station as a disc jockey during the day and as a play-by-play high school sports announcer on Friday nights. I quickly found a position as a private duty nurse at one of the two local hospitals.

At first, Patrick thought I shouldn't work, that I should stay home and be a wife, like my mother had done. But I had been working since I was 12 and staying home was not appealing. I had trained as a nurse because I liked nursing. Besides, I knew that after the fire we would not be living in Indio very much longer. With the bowling alley gone and Patrick's folks having moved away, there was nothing for us in Indio. We had to leave. Indio was fun for a few months, but we both wanted to see more of the world than the high school football stadium broadcast booth on Friday nights and the movie at the Aladdin Theater on Saturday night. I've often wondered what would have happened if Patrick had stayed working as a disc jockey at KREO — 1400 on your AM radio dial — 250 watts of power — the only radio station in the whole valley at the time — and I had remained on the staff at the hospital.

Of course, we'll never know the answer to that question, but it is fun to wonder. I do know this for sure. Our lives would have been vastly different then they have been, had we stayed in Indio.

So, after several nights of serious discussion — as serious as you can be in your very early twenties — we decided that living in Indio the rest of our lives was not what either one of us cared to do. Forgive us, Indio, but we had adventures to experience which were not to be found in the dusty Coachella Valley.

A few weeks after our decision, on a cool evening in January, 1960, Patrick and I put all of our worldly possessions onto a big jet airplane and flew off to seek our fortune and find our fame in the new State of Hawaii. We were young, free of debt, filled with the excitement for our grand new adventure and very much in love. We were, after all, as we sped out over the dark Pacific Ocean, going to be completely dependent on each other for the first time in our short marriage.

Hawaii was fun. We both found jobs. Patsy as an RN at Kaiser Hospital in Waikiki while I joined the sales staff of KOOD Radio, a brand new AM station in the Ala Moana Shopping Center.

While neither one of us made very much money, we were young, we had our health, we had the sand, surf and sun of Hawaii, and we had each other.

We didn't know at the time just how much we were going to need the strength of that special love, that special bond, built during those wonderful days in Hawaii. Every new marriage needs a time to seek the common level of trust, patience and consideration. In Hawaii, without either family, without any old friends and with just each other, Patsy and I formed the foundation of what has enabled us to endure and grow in our marriage and, much more importantly, in our lives with each other. We didn't know it while we played and loved and worked in Hawaii, but we would need all that bonding, all that trust, all that ability to depend on each other in the days and years which lay ahead of us.

As we look back on them now, we each consider those early days spent together in Hawaii, at the very outset of our marriage, as critical to the success of our marriage. We both believe that those first two years in Hawaii allowed us to develop a reliance and a dependence on each other that would see us through the hard days ahead. If a couple is to become one, it's not accomplished at the altar when you say "I do" or when the marriage is consummated. It happens over a period of time, after you have survived a series of tests and trials. Only a few people ever really become so close that they can be considered married. Most, I believe, become some kind of legal roommate to their spouses.

For two years, as we worked hard at our jobs, played in the pounding surf, walked through the quiet rain forests and flooded taro fields of Oahu, we grew to know one another quite well and to love each other very deeply.

After all, when we married, we were practically strangers. But after two years together in the islands we were now mates, lovers and each other's best friend.

By 1962, I became restless and was able to convince Patsy that we needed to return to the mainland. Hawaii had been a grand adventure, but there were other adventures to be found in other places.

We would leave behind in Hawaii some new, lifetime friends like Jack and Janet Sanborn who had taken the newlyweds to their bosoms and became our island family.

Jack is gone now, but we still are able to enjoy Janet's company whenever we get back to the islands or when she comes to the mainland to visit her children and their families. Janet and Jack Sanborn will always have a special place in our hearts.

After a visit to both Santa Barbara to see my folks and a trip to Boulder City, Nevada to visit with Luke and Lillian Whalen, we settled in Reno, Nevada just long enough for Patsy to get pregnant.

You can't imagine just how happy I was when she told me early one morning at breakfast that I was to be a father. Later that same morning, on the only television station in northern Nevada, I proudly told the whole world.

Patsy's pregnancy was in the seventh month when I persuaded her that we had to return to Hawaii, if my television career was to advance. We probably wouldn't have moved back to the islands if she hadn't worked at Kaiser Hospital for two years. Having worked there, she was well acquainted with — and trusted — a couple of their obstetricians.

23

Our first child, our daughter Teresa (I've left out her middle name because she hates it so much) arrived in the early morning hours of September 12, 1962. I was a father.

My goodness, how I loved being a father, right from that very first day. I think being a father is the greatest feeling in the whole world. What I didn't love about becoming a father, however, was not being allowed to greet my new daughter when she arrived. I felt cheated and very much an outsider during the whole process. The trusted doctor that Patsy had known so well when she worked there turned out to be an insensitive, self-centered medical man who was more interested in getting the job done than in how his patients might feel.

During the birth of Teresa, Patsy was completely unconscious — solely for the doctor's personal convenience. I was kept just as far away, downstairs watching the sunrise, prevented from even being near the delivery room when our baby girl arrived.

Teresa, full term and weighing in at over eight pounds, was born a very sleepy baby — drugged by that insensitive clod of a doctor who insisted Patsy be asleep for the delivery. Our baby was so slow to respond that she had to be placed in an isolette for three days (that's an incubator they used to use for "premies" when they were in distress). When I first saw Teresa, over an hour after she was born, she was still blue.

My general distrust and universal dislike of most doctors probably began to develop that night in Hawaii as I walked alone on the sands of Waikiki while my first child, groggy from the heavy medication administered to her mother, was being pulled into the world from my unconscious partner by an insensitive medical mechanic.

When Teresa was two, one of our many moves took the three of us to the central California town of Bakersfield. I hated Bakersfield. It was hot in the summer and foggy in the winter. I didn't have one friend in Bakersfield — except Patrick, who was spending a lot of time at the television station or playing golf or running around at night with his buddies from the station.

In Bakersfield, I spent a lot of time alone with a small child. Because she was so bright, we had a wonderful time together. My heart always goes out to all the mothers who need to return to work before their children are in school. They should be allowed to stay home with their child, if at all possible, even if it means fewer luxuries.

One night Patrick apparently was home, it seems. The moon and I both being in the right phase, our second child was conceived late in 1964.

Following Teresa's arrival, Patsy and I had agreed that we were not going to let the medical world put us, or our baby, through that terrible experience of being banned from the delivery room — Patsy asleep and me outside — as we had been in Hawaii. The next time — if we were lucky enough to have another child — we would both be there to welcome our baby into the world.

Now, here we were in Bakersfield, faced with the arrival of that

24

second child. It was time to test our resolve.

The first thing Patsy did was to select an obstetrician who agreed that both parents should be there to welcome their baby. He also thought that all those drugs were bad for both the mother and the baby.

He said it was "just fine with him" if the father wanted to be in the delivery room. I would, however, have to go through proper channels to get the formal permission of the hospital administration.

"It is, after all, their delivery room isn't it?"

No, I thought, it wasn't their delivery room. It was ours. While we weren't going to keep it, we were sure going to rent the exclusive use of it, at an outrageous cost, for a very short period of time. The exclusive use of it — no other patients were going to be disturbed or placed in any jeopardy. We were going to be in there alone. Didn't that make it ours? At least for the time being? I never have understood all the excuses which are so often put forward by doctors — and even by some nurses — about the propriety of their doing what they do in isolation. I find that much of it is very self serving.

In Bakersfield, in 1965, there were only two hospitals, the city owned Bakersfield General Hospital and the Catholic hospital, St. Mary's.

At that time Patsy and I were still Catholics, so I headed for St. Mary's to meet with a nun who served as the assistant administrator of the hospital. The good Sister had agreed to hear, and to consider, my reasons for asking the hospital to set aside their no fathers in the delivery room rule. I was sure my arguments would prevail.

The Sister was a very gentle woman. I remember she was soft spoken and seemed, at first, to be sympathetic to my desire to share the special moment of my child's arrival with my wife. She listened carefully, giving me her full attention — even though we were having this very private discussion in a corner of the hospital's busy lobby.

Finally, after hearing my well thought out and carefully prepared argument, the Sister said, "I'm sorry. It's a hospital rule which we are not allowed to break."

"What if I were a doctor, Sister. Would you allow me to be there if I were a doctor?"

"Oh, of course," she said.

"But I would be there as a father, not as a doctor, just like I want to be. Please, explain to me the difference."

"I'm sorry. It's just a rule that we can not break."

Trying desperately to maintain my respect for this devoted, religious lady, I asked the sixty-four dollar question. "Sister, do you have the power to make an exception to this silly rule or were you just being polite when you agreed to meet with me?"

"I was told to tell you that we were unable to make an exception to this rule," she said.

"No matter what I said? No matter how persuasive my argument? You came out here only able to say no. Is that correct?"

"I'm afraid it is, Mr. Nolan."

"Then, Sister, you're a phony. You gave me every reason to believe that I would be given a fair hearing. You lead me to believe that if I was able to present solid reasons for wanting to be there, you would consider allowing me to be present at the birth of my child. You have not only been dishonest with me, Sister, you've wasted my time and yours."

"I'm sorry," she said.

"Sorry? You should be ashamed of yourself, Sister."

I got up and walked out without another word. I'm sure she prayed for me that night.

The other hospital, the city owned hospital, was headed by a guy with a real Irish name, Sean something or other. Neither Patsy nor I can recall what it was — I wish I could, I'd like to give him some recognition in this book. I do recall that he was not a doctor, but an executive administrator.

Sean and I never met, except on the phone. It wasn't necessary that we meet, he said when I called for an appointment, he could tell me right there on the phone that I wasn't going to get by their, "no fathers allowed in delivery" hospital rule.

"However," he said, after hearing all my heartfelt reasons, "if we were ever going to make such an exception, you would be a perfect candidate."

Did I see a crack in his impenetrable stone wall?

While I wanted Patrick to be there for the birth of our child, I was not willing to do battle on the picket lines to see that he got there. I was sure that if there was a way, short of a frontal assault with a Sherman tank, that he would be there. I knew how strongly he felt about it, so I was relatively sure that he and I would share the birth of this child, but it was a battle he would have to wage on his own. I was determined that I was going to be there for the delivery, even if they were successful in keeping Patrick away. I wasn't about to wake up again and be told that I was a mother. I wanted to become a mother with my eyes open and my mind clear. I did agreed to a simple saddle block type of spinal, if it was needed, at the time of the delivery, but I did not want any general or sleep inducing drug.

Our doctor was still saying that he hoped Patrick was able to get permission to be with me. He was quite confident that Patrick wouldn't get that permission. Although the doctor had met Patrick on several of my prenatal visits, he didn't have a clue about Patrick's persistence.

In truth, all the doctor had to say to the hospital was that in his considered, medical opinion, Patrick needed to be there when our child was born. That simple "doctor's order" would have given the hospital a perfect reason to let down the drawbridge, without opening the flood gates. Flood gates which were, several years later, swung wide open by fathers like Patrick who insisted on being part of the birth process. But in 1965, in Bakersfield, Patrick was swimming upstream.

As the time for the baby approached I was working as a radio advertising time salesmen for KLYD, a daytime radio station in Bakersfield. My boss was a fellow named Dwight Case who kept telling me and the rest of the salesmen that he'd fire us if he caught us playing golf on "his" time. I was the top salesman on the staff and I played 18 holes almost every day that year. My handicap was seven. (Just thought you'd like to know, Dwight.)

I was playing golf with John Ogden, another salesman at KLYD, the day the baby was scheduled to arrive. When we wandered home about four in the afternoon, Patsy told us that she had started into labor a few hours before. It was Sunday, June 6, 1965, the twentieth anniversary of D-Day.

My D-Day with the hospital would be in the early hours of the next morning, as Patsy labored to bear our second child.

John and Patsy sat down and worked on the Sunday paper's crossword puzzle for a couple of hours. We knew there was no need to rush off the the hospital, so while Pats and John worked on twenty-six across and seventeen down, I went into the bedroom and took a nap because I knew we were in for a long, sleepless night, once serious labor began.

Years later, during the days when I searched for something or someone to blame for what was happening to Michele, I remembered standing at our kitchen sink in Bakersfield, doing the dishes. As I looked out across the vast agricultural fields of Kern County, I watched airplane after airplane swoop down and dump its load of toxic chemicals on the tender, young plants in those fields. It wasn't until years later, struggling to save Michele's life, that I recognized that those same agricultural crop dusters were also dumping load after load of toxic chemicals into my body and into the body of my as yet unborn child. Industrial apologists will tell you that there is no way anyone can prove that those chemicals were responsible for Michele's cancer. By the same token, they can't prove they weren't responsible, either.

Couple that with the fact that I grew up in the forties and fifties only a hundred miles from the atomic testing grounds in Nevada and you have all kinds of interesting possibilities for what may — or may not — have caused Michele's cancer.

Now, as I sat there in the dining room on Sunday afternoon, doing crossword in the kitchen with John, I knew this night was going to be a long night. A long, tiring night of labor, but I was prepared for it. I had been taking my vitamins and exercising.

That morning the nesting instincts must have been very strong. I had scrubbed and waxed the kitchen and the bathroom floors, vacuumed and dusted the whole house and finished three loads of laundry. I ran out of gas before I could finish all the windows.

My doctor had given me a couple of special exercises that would help ease the delivery and help my body return to normal after the birth. He hadn't actually provided me with a natural childbirth course of exercises, but what he had given me helped a great deal. I didn't know everything I should have known about a natural delivery, but I did know that with the heat we had that summer in Bakersfield, I was more than ready to deliver this child into the world.

Since the hospital had no prohibition against visitors being in the private labor rooms, Patrick was right there with me in our windowless cell from the start. He, unfortunately, smoked in those days, so every hour or so he'd go out to the waiting room where the other fathers were sitting, to have a cigarette. By ten o'clock in the evening he wasn't going out to have any more cigarettes. He was too busy. But he did go out a couple of times to call the administrator to press his case for being in the delivery room. Patrick wasn't about to give up.

I really believe that he wanted their permission, but I also know that he was prepared to break the rule at the point when no one could do anything about it — the point when I was ready to present this child. I didn't want a hassle, but I knew he felt very strongly about being with me through the entire birthing process, so I was prepared for almost anything. However, under the circumstances, I wasn't wasting a lot of my time worrying about it. I had my own job to do that night and Patrick had his.

About ten-thirty, after several attempts, I spoke to the guy who ran the hospital when he finally returned my call. I think he was feeling warm and relaxed because he was a lot friendlier than he had been when I had talked to him in his office. He was very patient, but remained firm.

If, he said, they let me in, it would open the floodgates and every father would want to be there and the hospital just couldn't allow that to happen.

Allow that to happen? Allow that to happen? Where are fathers supposed to be when they become parents? Fathers, as we have learned since those caveman days between the thirties and the mid sixties, have their own very important job to do doing this miraculous event called childbirth.

At this point in my life, as I write this, I have been present at the birth of four children — two were mine — and each time I am thrilled again by the absolute and utter magic of it all. The birth of a baby is an amazing, beautiful and wondrous thing to experience.

If you're a father-to-be, get educated! There are now hundreds of books on the subject. And get into the game — as a player. You will always remember that day. If you do nothing else in your life, be there when the mother of your child gives birth to your baby. There is no other moment like that available in life. It's as close as you can come to the feeling of pure joy. Pure joy!

That night in 1965, as we waited for Michele to move along the birth canal, the hospital administrator admonished me, "But what if, God forbid, something were to go wrong and we were to lose your wife, or the child?"

"That's just another one of those inane hospital excuses, Sean. If we were in an automobile crash and Patsy was dying, do you think I would accept being told to walk a few yards down the highway until she was dead?

"Where the hell do I belong if she dies, Sean? I belong there, with her. And if the child dies or is not normal, don't you think I should be there to help Patsy bear that burden? What can you possibly be thinking about when you come up with these self-serving reasons to prevent people from doing what they should be doing?," I demanded.

I was tired, running out of patience and getting steamed. Sean wasn't even listening to me. He knew I was right, but he was too proud or too scared of the hospital board to admit it and get the hell out of my way.

Finally, after about twenty minutes of fairly forceful discussions on my part, I said, "Listen, Sean, I'm going back to Patsy, where I belong right now. And I'm not going to leave her. I'm going to be with her when this baby's born, period. And there really isn't a whole hell of a lot you can do about it, short of calling out the damn Marines. I will not go quietly into that dark waiting room, Sean. Now, why don't you make it easy on everybody, particularly the nurses and other members of the staff here, to say nothing of my wife, our baby and me, and get the hell out of our way?"

A light must have gone off in his head when I said that. I guess what I said finally helped him understand just how important this was to us. I also think he was convinced that I'd be a royal pain in the butt if he did try to stop me, physically.

He didn't want to back down, but he saw it was better to give in a little and thereby avoid dealing with a completely crazed father.

So, reluctantly, he finally said, "OK, if you'll put on a gown and mask, I'll let you stand in the doorway of the delivery room. I'll go that far with you, but keep it to yourself."

"Stand in the doorway? Right!" I said, under my breath.

The war was over.

Then he said, "Tell the head nurse that I said it was OK, if you put on a gown and a mask."

"No!" I said, "You tell her. I don't want there to be any question that it's you on the phone and that you're giving me the go ahead to gown and mask and bend the hospital's precious rules. And, thanks, Sean."

Since I had taken his call at the nurses station and all the nurses were standing there listening to me with their mouths open, I just handed the head nurse the phone, winked, and walked back to the labor room, smiling. We'd won.

I knew that once I was in the basic greens, I was on the team. That "stand in the doorway" business meant nothing once I was dressed in the team's colors. By this time the nurses were all in favor of my being there.They had all seen how well I was working with Patsy as the contractions washed over her. They knew I was making their jobs a lot easier and they saw how important it was to both Patsy and to me for us to share this wonderful experience. I wasn't in the way, I was on the team, playing a positive and important role.

One nurse, the one who was especially assigned to us, had been very cooperative and not at all threatened by our efforts to break the normal routine. She seemed to understand what being together for this birth meant to us and she was very much on our side. I'm sorry that neither one of us can remember her name, but if she's reading this, she may remember us and smile, knowing that we still remember her gentle bedside manner and thoughtfulness, even if we can't recall her name. So, if you are reading this, and if you were working in the maternity section of Bakersfield Memorial Hospital on the morning of June 7, 1965, thanks for your help. We may not remember your name, but we will never forget your wonderful support and your tender loving care.

Happy as Patrick was when he came back into the labor room with his news, our all night adventure was not quite over yet. We still had to have this baby.

Sometime in the middle of the night, Patrick ran out of patience with me and my slow labor. It was probably around three or four in the morning. He just wanted to get this over with. He was tired, cranky and, as the hours dragged on, was being less and less of a labor coach. He was making me mad as hell at him. His lack of patience made me feel like he thought I was holding back this kid, just to piss him off. The nurses all told him to get some sleep. I told him to take a hike.

Finally, he did take a break for an hour or so and went out for a walk. He needed to be a parent again, but so did I. I was very happy to have him get out of there for a while. I was doing the best I could. It was just taking a long time to move this child along the birth canal and out to the bright, new world. Unfortunately, Patrick thought it should take less time than my body intended to take with the process.

That night, Patrick was not getting his way and he was acting like a spoiled brat about it. There have been times, and this was one of them, when I have wanted to bop him for acting like that.

At about seven-thirty in the morning, my doctor appeared in the doorway to see how things were going. Patrick wasn't very friendly. He knew that the doctor had just finished enjoying a full night's sleep.

While Patrick was tired and just about out of gas, the doctor, on the other hand, was all rested and chipper.

As to how things were going with me, things had almost stopped. I was spent, the contractions had slowed to a tight squeeze now and then and I was getting nowhere with this baby. I was also nearly bushed from the battle.

A new staff of nurses had come on duty at seven. We were sorry to see the eleven to seven shift depart, because they had become our friends, during the night.

The new gang was full of energy and eager to be of service. Our "new" nurse was just doing what she normally did when she suggested that Patrick might want to step outside of the labor room while the doctor examined me.

Patrick shot a wicked glare up at her and snapped, "No, thanks. I know what's under those sheets. How the hell do you think she got in this condition?"

The doctor raised his hand, indicating that it might be better for everyone to just leave Patrick alone and get on with the things that needed to be done. I was very relieved. Patrick was ready to tear a piece out of someone and I didn't have the strength to intercede on behalf of the person he might select. I also didn't want to lose the support of our nurse.

After his examination, the doctor told us that he thought the problem was that the my membranes had not yet ruptured. He said that if he gave me a little help we might move this labor along a little faster. What he proposed to do was to take a long clamp and tear a hole in the wall of the amniotic sack to let out the water. Then the baby could move out and down the birth canal. I had worked all night with almost no results. It was very discouraging. I was ready to give up. The clamp business was a completely painless procedure which took about ten seconds, producing, as it should, a gush of amniotic fluid and then, within seconds, one terrific contraction.

"Oh, my! Hang on. Here we go," I said through gritted teeth.

"There," said the doctor, "that should get things moving now. You keep working and I'll be back in a hour or so to see how things are going. You're doing just fine, Patsy."

The doctor left to take his dog to the vet, leaving us, once again, alone together in our little windowless cell.

To say that the action picked up after that would be, at the very least, a serious understatement. Within minutes, my labor pains — the contractions — returned in full force. As they gained in intensity, grew in length and came closer together, I knew it wouldn't be long before this child would be with us.

Patrick's interest in what we were doing, returned in full force too, as did his enthusiasm. He seemed filled with a renewed strength, seeing as I did, a whole new dynamic return to the labor of childbirth. He said later that he suddenly felt rested, wide awake, alert and filled with new energy — and a new calm. The summit was finally in sight and we were racing toward it together. Every ninety seconds or so, the three of us took another giant leap forward.

Patrick's firm encouragement, his tender touch with a cool cloth on my head — along with his rediscovered excitement — eased my anxiety.

I got busy meeting each contraction with all the concentration I could muster. Patrick, the baby and I were now in perfect rhythm. After about twenty minutes of very hard work I knew that the baby had completed transition and was ready to burst into the world. I could feel the baby's head forcing my legs apart. I told Patrick to look and confirm that the signals which my body was sending up to my brain were, indeed, correct. Had the baby crowned?

"I can see the top of the head," he said with a controlled excitement, "We're about to be parents again, babe."

Patrick stuck his head out of our little labor room and called calmly to our nurse, "We're about to have a baby. I think it's time to move."

"Are you sure?," she asked.

"Absolutely. Give me a hand with the bed," Patrick said. He was in total control of his emotions, the situation and, it seemed, the event.

The nurse didn't even bother to check the position of the baby herself. Trusting by now that he knew what he was talking about, she just grabbed the other end of the bed as another nurse pushed the door to the labor room to the full open position. We were on our way.

With Patrick pushing the head of the bed, they pulled me toward the empty delivery room which was only a few feet away.

"See if the doctor is back in the hospital, yet, please," the nurse instructed a colleague.

As they wheeled me through the door, Patrick asked where to find the clean gowns and the masks.

"I don't want to break any rules around here," he said with just the slightest hint of sarcasm in his voice.

Everyone, including me, smiled. Patrick's eyes were dancing with excitement and anticipation. Walter Mitty was, at last, in his glory — a full fledged member of the obstetrical team.

One of the nurses held a gown open for him to slip into as another pulled a surgical mask down over his head. He was on the team, suited up in a lovely shade of green and ready to play.

The nurses were very proud of him. They knew he belonged there with me. As they were busy welcoming this new father-to-be to the maternity staff, they'd completely forgotten about the one who was there to deliver the baby.

Laying on the edge of the bed, looking down at a gap between the bed and the delivery table, I felt sure that during the next contraction, I was going to wind up on that cold, hard floor. But, in just a few seconds, they all returned their attention to me as quickly as they had abandoned me.

With Patrick's help they eased me across that awful gap onto the freezing delivery table. The instant they slid me over onto the plastic cover on the delivery table, I almost had the baby, because that icy table was a completely unexpected shock to my warm, bare bottom. Boy, was that table cold.

Moments later, as Patsy was still fussing about how cold the table was, the doctor returned from the vet and stuck his head in the door.

"How're we doing in here?" he asked in a completely relaxed, unhurried manner.

Our nurse, who had seen the crown of the baby's head by now and knew we had just minutes before presentation, turned toward him and barked some very succinct orders.

"Don't bother to change, Doctor. You don't have time. Get in here, right now. I've got everything ready. Just get a gown and mask on. We're having a baby here, and we're having it right now," she said, leaving no room for comment or discussion, much less disagreement.

Off came the coat and tie and on went a mask, gown and gloves. He'd almost missed out on all the fun.

As I encouraged Patsy to relax, the team, now working in perfect sync, rolled Patsy toward me onto her left side while I pulled her up into a tight ball. The doctor was preparing to slide a big needle between two of her lower vertebrae, injecting a small dose of a numbing agent known as a saddle block. They call it that because the part of the body that it affects is the part that touches a saddle when you're riding a horse. But this was no canter in the country. We were having a baby.

In later years, we learned just how ineffective that type of anesthesia is during late stages of a woman's delivery. The hard pains have passed with transition and the pressure applied by the baby's head has, by now, almost completely deadened the nerves at the end of the vaginal opening. The saddle block, at that point, is usually more psychological than practical. it also provides anesthesia for the episiotomy.

As the needle entered her spinal column, I held her very tightly, curled up in my arms in as tight a knot as her large belly would allow.

"Just hold very, very still and don't move, my love," I whispered in her ear.

She did what she was told to do, perfectly. It was over in a few seconds.

We rolled Patsy over onto her back and raised her legs into the delivery table stirrups. She was sweating like a mule, but completely relaxed and perfectly calm. She had done her job and she knew it. The rest would take only a little more effort on her part. The delivery of this new human being would go very quickly now. Most of it was in the catching, not in the pushing.

I took a wet cloth and wiped her forehead. She welcomed the coolness with a loving look as our eyes met. I was so very proud of her.

As the doctor pulled his little stool up to the foot of the table, he realized that there was another masked member on his team.

He looked up at me, positioned beside Patsy's head at the end of the table, and as our eyes met, said, "How'd you pull this off?"

He was very surprised to see that I was able to break security to be there in the delivery room, the last place he thought he'd ever see me.

"Salesmanship."

The eyes of the nurses were all smiling behind their little surgical masks. I was grinning from ear to ear under mine. Patsy slapped me playfully on the arm and almost laughed out loud. One of the nurses moved a large mirror out of the corner of the room and positioned it just over the doctor's shoulder.

"Let me know when you can see," she said to Patsy. Patsy and I would welcome our new baby into the world in the mirror — watching this miraculous event together.

After a small incision, called an episiotomy, the baby's head slipped easily into the doctor's large hand.

"Can everyone see?"

We both said we could see as we watched a new little life make its way into the light. It was the most amazing thing I had ever seen.

As the next contraction began, the baby rolled on its side, gently slipping from the cocoon of her mother's womb into the doctor's gloved hands.

"It's a little girl!" announced the doctor as he confidently wiped her face and raised her onto Patsy's tummy.

Patsy sat partly upright. With one corner of the green drape she gently wiped away a few of the little drops of nature's lubricant which coated the tiny face of this new human creature.

One minute we were two laboring adults, one working the female muscles that would advance the delivery of her baby, the other offering encouragement, asking her to focus her attention on the job at hand and softly reassuring her that she could climb to the summit of this massive peak.

One minute we were holding each other's hands very tightly, just two people in a room with a few strangers… and then, suddenly, Michele Kathleen Nolan was with us.

Light blue at first and then, as her lungs filled with air for the first time, she quickly turned pale pink, then rosy red. She was a bright,

healthy baby girl. One minute we were all bearing down and intense...
and then, suddenly, she was with us, gurgling and blinking in the bright
lights of the delivery room. And all was right with the world.

As soon as she was released from the lifeline she no longer needed,
Michele Kathleen was wrapped in a soft blanket and handed to Patsy. I
couldn't help it. I reached out and touched a tiny, uncovered foot. It was
Michele's first, ungloved, human touch. I'm still very proud that I was
the one to give her that first touch.

Little did we know what a tremendous impact this seven pound,
fourteen ounce little girl would have on us, on our family and on our
lives, in the years ahead.

The rest was routine. Washing the baby, cleaning up the mother,
congratulating the father and transporting me to my cool, bright hospital
room. It had been one terrific morning.

Before we left the delivery room area, Patrick thanked each of the
nurses, personally. Two of them kissed him goodbye. As a member of
the team, he'd pulled his share of the load.

Before we left the delivery room, Patrick, his eyes filled with tears of
joy, leaned down and gently kissed me. He was very proud of what I
had done. We were extremely close to each other at that moment. We
had been there for each other, when it counted. What I saw in his eyes,
was so eloquent and so loving.

However, as soon as I got to my room, I was suddenly very tired.
The adrenalin was quickly draining from my veins and the long night of
labor was starting to take effect. I told Patrick to go home, take a bath,
rest, call our parents and tell Teresa that she had a beautiful little sister.
All I wanted to do right now was go to sleep for two days. Even the
shot they gave me to help shrink my womb wouldn't prevent me from
sleeping. I'd climbed to the summit, and with Patrick's help, I had
planted our flag on top of the world. Now it was time for me to rest.

Patrick kissed me again and slipped out the door. He was grinning
from ear to ear as I watched him dance down the hallway toward the
exit. You'd have thought he had a full night's rest.

I learned from the car radio, on the way home, that during the time
our new little Gemini, Michele, was being relieved of her umbilical cord in
Memorial Hospital in Bakersfield, Ed White was making America's first
space walk at the end of his own umbilical cord outside the Gemini 4
spaceship in space, miles above our heads. That scorched capsule sits
today on the ground floor of the Air & Space Museum at the
Smithsonian Institution in Washington, D.C.

In 1974, exactly nine years later, on her birthday, Michele actually
got to touch that Gemini 4 space capsule during a family visit to the
nation's capitol. I'm sure that seeing Michele with that Gemini capsule
meant more to me than it did to her. Michele, as you will learn, is not
easy to impress.

The first thing I did when I got home from the hospital the day
Michele was born was to retrieve Teresa from the neighbor's where she
had spent the night. She was very happy to learn that we had produced

34

a girl named Michele and not a little boy named Patrick. She really wanted a little baby sister.

I called both sets of grandparents, then fixed Teresa (whom I've always called Charlie) a little breakfast.

I was still sitting somewhere up there in space with Ed White on cloud nine when I said, "Charlie," smoothing back a lock of her hair, "your momma sure does make beautiful babies."

"Yeah, Dad. I know," she said with her usual self confidence.

For three years, there had been just two of us, then for another three plus years, it was just the three of us, Charlie, Patsy and me...

... and then, suddenly, Michele Kathleen was with us, and we would never, ever be the same again.

At four one morning our phone rang.
It was Patrick's mother saying that his dad was very ill. Mom was scared
and anxious and had gotten out of bed and gone down to the business to call
Patrick so his dad wouldn't hear how worried she was over his illness.
The days ahead would not easy ones for any of us.

Chapter Two

Three Years of Ups & Downs and Then Dad!

When Michele was only 4 months old, we left Bakersfield for the television mecca of the west coast, Los Angeles, The City of Angels. There, Patrick happily joined the Metromedia station, KTTV, channel 11. He was very excited about being a television director in a major television market, at last.

After about six months at KTTV, Patrick was asked to join the staff of The Joe Pyne Show, a nationally syndicated radio and television talk show series. His star was ascending. I was very proud of him.

Patrick was never home during the Pyne days. He booked the guests, arranged the schedule, produced and supervised the "live" recording of two ninety minute TV talk shows and twelve one hour talk radio programs each week. It was a killer of a schedule.

While Patrick was busy in the trenches of big time TV, I was busy with a couple of wonderful little girls. We spent time at the park, we cooked dinner for dad and we enjoyed our days together, reading and getting Teresa ready to start school the following a year.

Michele could be such a funny little kid. She went through a period of several months where she would only eat Cheerios, spaghetti and peanut butter and jelly sandwiches, period. One time she sat for fifteen minutes chewing a mouth full of beef stew and when I asked her to open her mouth the bite of stew was all still in there. It wasn't even bruised. She never was bratty about it, she just didn't eat it if it wasn't peanut butter and jelly, spaghetti or a bowl of Cheerios.

Finally, I stopped getting upset about it. I figured that she was getting lots of protein, milk, bread and a few vegetables in the jelly and the spaghetti sauce. Since I was able to slip a banana into the cereal once in a while and from time to time I could get her to drink some orange juice, I figured she was being well fed.

Right in the middle of our second year in L.A., Patrick's dad, Patrick Nolan, the elder, suddenly became very seriously ill. His mom called at four one morning to say that she was scared to death that dad might be dying.

Patrick told his mom to bring dad to L.A., immediately, so we could get him to the best doctors we could find.

The doctor dad had been seeing in the little town of Indio just kept guessing about what was wrong with him. It was another case of a doctor who was afraid to admit he "don't have all the answers." This particular doctor, instead of admitting he didn't know what was wrong with dad, had told him he was probably just having trouble shaking the flu. By then, dad had been trying to shake the flu for three months. It was long past time to do something else.

While mom and dad were packing for the trip, Patrick called a young surgeon, Tom Humphreys, who had been a guest expert on the Pyne show a few weeks before. Patrick had quite liked Tom.

It was nearly five in the morning, but Tom Humphreys not only called us right back, he called Indio and talked to dad for over thirty minutes about his history, his symptoms and his feelings.

Before seven o'clock that morning, Tom called and arranged to have dad see his colleague, Dr. Harold Strick, an internist, later that day.

We were all scared to death because dad was just never, ever sick. But we were fairly confident because we felt that we were dealing with two terrific physicians who cared. It turned out that we were right about them both. They were great physicians, good doctors and good people. And they both cared deeply for their patients.

I almost collapsed when I walked in to the living room and took a look at my dad. His eyes were just dark circles, sunken back in his head. His color was not that of a living person. He was slate gray and he looked scared. Dad seemed to sense that he was deathly ill.

Not normally a man who was easily frightened, Dad was scared because he didn't know what was killing him. I'd had a knot in my stomach since Mom called that morning, and now I felt it tighten another notch.

My dad was in big trouble and everyone in the family looked to me for answers. My mom's look was almost desperate. She knew that the Indio doctor was bluffing, but she was scared that dad might be beyond help by now. She had given me no idea, until four this morning, that my dad was as sick as he obviously was as he sat there looking to me to do what he knew he was now unable to do for himself.

I went to him and put my arms around him as he sat there in the chair in the living room.

"It's going to be all right now, Dad. Don't worry. We're going to take care of you."

I kissed him and wiped away my own tears. I was just as scared as he was. The traditional roles of father and son were being reversed.

Patrick took Dad to see Hal Strick while I stayed home with mom and the girls. Three hours later, Patrick finally called. He was at the hospital, admitting his father for tests and observation.

After examining his father, Hal Strick said, "I don't know what's wrong with Dad, but whatever it is, it's killing him, Patrick. We've got to hurry up and find out what it is before it's too late."

That damned Indio doctor had used up several weeks of precious time pretending that he was taking good care of Dad, when, in fact, he didn't have the slightest clue as to what was wrong with the man. That stupid, vain doctor had stubbornly refused to admit he didn't know what was wrong with Dad, hoping instead that whatever it was would just go away. It didn't, of course.

We didn't have that problem with dad's doctors in L.A. Hal Strick and Tom Humphreys were completely candid with us from the first moment.

They didn't know what the problem was, and they said so. But they were also doing all they could to find out what was killing my dad. They'll always have our admiration and our complete respect, both as physicians and as people.

Patrick was dividing his days between the studio — where he was still trying to keep up with that killer schedule — and the hospital where his dad was going down hill every day. It was killing Patrick to watch his father slipping away and not be able to do anything to change it. Over the years, Patrick had grown accustomed to being in charge of things, but this was something he could not control, could not manage, could not direct. The disease was in control and Patrick was suffering from the frustration of not being able to get a handle on even what it was, much less how to control its deadly advances.

My days were divided between work and frequent visits to the hospital, but my nights were spent at home with the girls because Dad wanted Patsy to be his special duty night nurse. She spent every one of the forty-seven nights he was in that hospital at his bedside — all night long.

Dad was dying and not being able to stop it was killing Patsy, too. While Dad was suffering a great deal, his special duty nurse was suffering her own personal pain. She loved Dad very much. I'll never know how she held up for those seven terrible weeks, alone, each night — all night, with my dad, as she watched him slowly, painfully die.

These days were vastly important days for Patsy and me. Days which would prepare us for the tests yet to come. With Dad, we were dealing, as best we could, with a mutual challenge. The illness of my father was the first big test of our strength as a couple — a married couple. As we fought to save my dad's life, we did it in concert. We held each other when the pain got too intense. We supported each other when our energy was sapped. We looked to each other for the strength we each needed to face another day of IVs, tubes, machines, blood tests, new dressings and the unstoppable advance of the mysterious disease that was killing Dad.

Dad may have been dying, but in our struggle to help him, Patsy and I were building layers of dependency on the other and trust in each other. I hated watching, helplessly as my father died, but I recognized that my pain was eased just by the very presence of my special partner. I don't know if I could have survived those terrible weeks without Patsy's tremendously important place in my heart and at Dad's side.

Dad's case became a cause for everyone at Sunset Hollywood Hospital. The entire hospital, from the doctors and nurses to the x-ray technicians, were going crazy trying to discover what was killing my father. My dad had always had a special way of touching people.

They did an exploratory operation after six days of tests and x-rays and found a mass of tissue in his abdomen that none of the labs was able to identify.

They called in cancer specialists, kidney guys, blood experts and anyone else they could think of to look at the charts and the records and the tests and the x-rays. Dad was dying and they didn't seem to be able to change things.

They didn't know what was killing him, and they admitted it. But, admitting it didn't help, we all just wanted to save dad's life, or at the very least, find out what the hell we were fighting.

In the middle of our struggle with dad's mysterious, deadly illness, I got into a hassle on the phone with a minor, mid-level, junior executive in the programming department of KTTV. As the conversation quickly went down hill he told me that he was giving me my notice.

I told him, pointedly, "You really are something. Before you fire someone it's incumbent on you to find out if they actually work for you. How can you fire me, Al? I don't work for you. Now, if you'll excuse me, I'm going to the hospital and feed Dad his lunch."

I hung up and drove the seven blocks to the hospital to see my dad.

Although I was the Associate Producer of The Joe Pyne shows, I wasn't totally aware of the contractual arrangement between The Production Center at Metromedia, where we produced the television shows, and the company I was employed by, Hartwest, the New York based syndicator. Metromedia, I discovered, held all the cards. So, when I got back from the hospital they had pulled my gate pass. I wasn't allowed on the studio lot. I not only couldn't I get past the guard gate, I couldn't get into my office and I couldn't work on the shows. They play rough in tinsel town. In less than two hours I was on the street — an unemployed civilian. I decided to take all of them before the bar of justice, a decision which turned out to be one of the biggest mistakes of my life.

Not only was his dad dying of an unknown ailment, but Patrick had now been summarily kicked out of the best job he had had up to that point in his career. And all over a silly fight with a lightweight assistant program guy. It was a tough time for my husband, but the problem of his dad's illness was really the only thing that mattered to either of us at that time.

First there had been the surgery, then, a day later, Dad went into shock when his adrenal glands shut down. Then he developed very painful stomach ulcers .

By the time Patrick was so rudely dumped at the Pyne Show, his dad was in intensive care. He had been rushed back into emergency surgery, having perforated a stomach ulcer.

Apparently, he had developed the ulcers as a result of the the medication we were giving him to balance his adrenal system.

While I was spending the nights with Dad, Patrick would come in every morning at dawn and stay with him throughout the day, dividing his time between his dad and giving what comfort he could to his mom. Patrick had a lot on his shoulders during those terrible days.

One morning, almost without warning, Dad slipped into a coma. I think his body was trying to hide from the pain. At first, he was able to communicate with us by squeezing our hand — one squeeze for yes, two for no.

Even though his eyes were open, they wandering aimlessly, unfocused and uncontrolled. Each day we knew the coma was deepening. After a few days in the coma, the hand squeezes grew weaker and weaker.

One morning, Patrick came in early, as usual. I was sitting on the bed, holding dad's hand, gently talking to him, gently stroking back the strands of thin hair on his head. We were alone, just Dad and I. The other nurses were all busy with other patients there in the Intensive Care Unit.

Patrick leaned over and kissed his dad as he asked me, "Are you able to get through to him at all, Pats?" (Pats is his special name for me. Patrick and our friend, Walt Baker, are the only ones who call me that.)

I touched his shoulder, kissed him and replied, "Not for several hours, honey. I think he's slipped farther away during the night. He won't squeeze my hand now at all. The last time I had a squeeze was sometime around midnight."

Patrick took his dad's other hand, smoothed back a strand of hair from his dad's forehead with his other hand and quietly said, "Good Morning, Dad. I love you."

At that moment, a very extraordinary thing happened.

Patrick's dad closed his eyes for just a second. It was the first time he had shown any control over them in days. When he opened them, his eyes were perfectly still. He was looking — actually focusing his eyes — on his son's face. It must have taken an enormous force of sheer will power for him to do that.

Dad held his gaze, his eyes perfectly steady for a full eight or ten seconds, looking directly into Patrick's eyes. Then, calmly, his eyes closed again and when they opened a second later, they were once again wandering, completely out of control. He was back on the other side. For a few seconds, neither of us spoke.

"Honey," I said to Patrick, "he just told you goodbye."

Patrick gently wiped away a tear that was rolling slowly down his dad's cheek. Letting his own tears fall onto the bed, he softy said to me, "I know, Pats. I know."

Several days later Dad needed help breathing so we elected to let them do a tracheotomy. That may have been a mistake. We weren't going to change anything and this procedure was just going to prolong my father's long agony. But we were still hoping for a miracle.

The next afternoon all the players were gathered around Dad's bed.

Krista, a young blond ICU nurse who had taken Dad to her heart and who, like so many others in that small hospital, had practically become a member of our family, was there.

Hal Strick, the only one of dad's doctors who had made a personal visit to see him every single day Dad was in the hospital — 47 of them by now — was there, as well.

My mom, who had married Dad when she was still a teenager and who was now losing her lifetime partner and best friend, was at his side for the last time.

Patsy, who by now wasn't bothering to go home at all, was standing next to mom, with her arm around her shoulders, still trying to comfort her family as best anyone could as those last few hours of my father's life slipped away from us.

"Hal, let's see how he does breathing on his own, without the respirator," I said.

Hal nodded at her and Krista gently removed the plastic hose from the tracheotomy tube that had been inserted into dad's windpipe. When she took it off, Dad continued to breath on his own. He only took slow, shallow breaths, but they were unassisted. He was in a deep coma, but he was still able to breath on his own, at least a little.

The room was silent for a moment, as we listened to those labored breaths from my dad.

"Krista," I said quietly, but firmly, "Unplug that thing from the wall and don't plug it back in, no matter who tells you to do so."

The words came out of me with a strong, sure strength that I have never regretted. It was the right thing to do. I knew it at the time and I still know it today, over twenty-seven years later. My father's courageous, painful battle for life was finally going to come to an end, unassisted. It just wasn't fair to ask him to go any further.

Hal Strick, who was standing beside me, put his arm around my shoulders and said, "Don't ever let anyone tell you that was the wrong thing to do, Patrick. It's time to let him go, and you're the right one to do it. I'm deeply sorry, my friend. Your father was a fine man."

I'll always love Hal Strick for what he did for Dad and for giving Patrick such wonderful support at that critical moment in our lives.

Hal's a very special physician, who hates losing any patient, but he knew that we had done the best we could do. He also knew we had lost. He knew that Dad had fought the good fight, but he also knew, as Patrick and I instinctively seemed to know, that it was time to admit that we were beaten. We didn't know what it's deadly name was, yet, but we knew that the disease had won.

Dad lived for three hours after Patrick unplugged him. We were all with him when he just let out one, final, shallow breath and never took another one. He was only sixty-one years old when he died. And after forty-seven days of hell, he was finally at peace, free of the pain, free of the struggle.

When we left Los Angeles to go to Indio for the funeral, our house was in a complete shambles. I had been spending nights at the hospital and days sleeping. Patrick had been spending days at the hospital and nights sleeping. Our two very active daughters had been living in the midst of all the turmoil.

When we left for the funeral, I hired Vicki Cornalini, a teenage girl who lived next door, to clean the house while we were gone.

When we returned, the house was spotless from top to bottom, but in the middle of the living room floor was a 1918 Indian head penny. I still believe that it was my parting gift from Patrick's coin collecting father.

Three months after Dad died, Hal Strick called me one day and asked me if I could come by his home that evening. He had some news for me about dad's illness.

It seems that frozen sections of that strange mass they had removed from Dad during that exploratory operation had been sent to several pathology labs, both in L.A. and elsewhere in the country. One of the samples wound up in Washington, D.C. at the National Institute of Pathology. They couldn't identify it so they made it a special assignment for one of their researchers. They wanted to know what that tissue was. So, naturally, did we.

Now, after three months, we finally had the answer.

It seems that my dad had somehow contracted a very rare disease called, Nocardioses Astroidous. (It's so rare that it doesn't even have a "common" name.) It's a type of fungus that only kills about five people a year in the whole country. It's very rare. Dad's chances of being struck by lightening were far greater than getting killed by this stuff. All the medical world knows about it is covered on a single page in a big, thick medical book called Rare Diseases In Mankind.

There was some satisfaction in knowing, at long last, what had taken Dad from us, but I now I had to worry about feeding the family. I couldn't get a job in the L.A. broadcasting community. Taking Metromedia to court had been a terrible mistake. They're not only a very powerful group of people, but Los Angeles is a "company" town. The company had closed ranks and I was on the outside, unable to get back in.

Having filed a lawsuit against one of the nation's largest and most powerful communications companies, Patrick was finding it impossible to even get an appointment to talk to anyone in Hollywood, much less find a job.

Hartwest, his employer, had turned their collective backs on him, giving his job to a guy Patrick had brought in and trained. Metromedia made a dozen or so phone calls around town and the doors of television were effectively slammed in Patrick's face. It was a tough time for all of us.

One day Patrick answered an ad in Broadcasting Magazine and within a week or so he was off to Colorado to run a small town radio station. The long arm of Metromedia didn't, it seemed, reach quite everywhere.

The girls and I spent the next six weeks selling off stuff, packing and getting ready to move to Fort Morgan, Colorado.

We spent eight months on the eastern slope of the Rockies. I worked a few nights in the maternity section of the local hospital, helping deliver new little farm hands. Patrick was the station's only salesman, did all the high school play-by-play and delivered a morning and an evening sports report during the news. Along with the aging station owner, he ran the station and quickly became one of the town's best known citizens. Talk about a big fish in a little pond.

But the call of the big pond remained great. One afternoon, our old friend, Walt Baker, called us.

Did we want to come back to L.A?

There was a director's job open at the RKO station where Walter worked, KHJ-TV (Now, KCAL, channel 9). I started packing for our return to L.A. that very day.

So, back we went to Hollywood. I started out as the weekend news director and within three months was asked to produce the Emmy Award winning, weekday talk show, "Tempo."

43

"Tempo" was a very contemporary, live talk show in the sixties. It was the brain child of the station's brilliant Executive Producer, Milt Hoffman.

"Tempo" was a killer to produce. We had only seven people on the staff, producing four hours of rapid fire talk show segments, each day, five days a week — twenty hours of live television each week. (Today's "Donahue" has over forty people producing just five hours of programming a week.) The days were fourteen hours long and weekends were brief little islands of joy at the end of five days of Hoffman Hell.

We had Kings, Princes, and a few now and future Presidents on the show. Tramps, city slickers, authors and, because we were in Hollywood, a constant procession of stars and "wannabe" stars were booked, too.

During the eighteen months I worked on that show we had everybody from Vice President Hubert Humphrey to Gypsy Boots on the air, live.

"The Gipper," Ronald Reagan, who was the Governor of California at the time, was almost a regular. We interviewed him in his limo one day when there was a death threat on his life. We just drove the car right into the studio. "Tempo" was an exciting show. I loved doing it.

Teresa, Michele and I were busy settling into our, snug little home in Studio City. We had found a place with a nice fenced yard on a quiet street, just a block from the nearest freeway entrance.

There were trips to Disneyland, to the small village of Yucaipa to visit our friends Dale and Mildred Hudec and their five kids and excursions to the beach for a week with some friends. We enjoyed dinner with the Bakers, went to Dodger Stadium to watch Koufax and Drysdale pitch and even ran away to Mexico for four days without the girls. It was a nice time in our lives. We were healing from the loss of Patrick's dad, Patrick's career was back on track and Teresa and Michele were bringing lots of joy into our lives. We were a very happy family.

Happy, that is, until the evening of Thursday, November 14, 1968, the day our world exploded.

As Michele lay on the examining table that night,
you could see a swelling on her right side.
The doctor asked how long it had been there.
I had to admit that I had never seen it before.

Chapter Three

That Terrible Night & The Awful Day To Follow!

It was raining in Los Angeles on Thursday, November 14, 1968. I had worked at the studio well past the dinner hour, coming home tired and cranky from the extra heavy freeway traffic, the tough day, and the rain which always seems to confound the Los Angeles drivers.

As I came through the front door of our cozy little home in the San Fernando Valley, just up the freeway from Hollywood, I was still fussing over something at work and being just plain crabby about life in general.

Patsy had fed the girls earlier, keeping dinner for us warm in the oven. When I was late she usually waited and ate with me.

When I walked through the door, Patsy was sitting in the rocking chair, gently rocking three year old Michele. I didn't notice the serious look on my wife's face right away.

"What's up?" I asked, wondering what was for dinner.

Patsy, who doesn't over react to most situations, said, with just the slightest edge of concern in her voice, "Michele fell when the girls were getting ready for bed. Now she says her tummy won't stop hurting."

Michele had never been a whiner. When she would fall or trip, she'd just get up, dust herself off, and go on with what she was doing. She never complained, or fussed, for very long. But this time she had continued to cry about what seemed like a minor incident. She complained of a pain in her tummy that wouldn't go away.

The fact that Patsy was worried caused me more concern than anything else at that moment. Patsy doesn't panic or get overly concerned about the normal bumps and bruises encountered during childhood. But there are times her sixth sense can be fine particularly acute. I've learned to pay close attention to that sensitivity.

"Do you think she really hurt herself, Pats?"

"I'm not sure. She never cries for more than a few seconds when she gets hurts. It's been almost an hour since she fell. And she only fell a few inches, off of the bed, onto Teresa. I really am beginning to get a little concerned. She seems to be having a hard time breathing, too. Maybe it's just her cold," she said, trying to talk herself into believing that she was on the verge of letting this incident get out of perspective.

Suffering from an early winter cold, Michele had been to see the pediatrician just the day before. She was still pretty stuffy, so the crying had succeeded in filling her chest and throat with lots of congestion.

"If you think it's more than just a hard fall or a bump, let's call the doctor," I said.

Much to my surprise and without another word, Patsy, got up, handed me the baby and went to the phone.

I was now sure that Patsy was a a great deal more worried than I had first thought. Patsy never cries wolf. Apparently she just wanted to have me reassure her that she wasn't being overly concerned about wanting to call the doctor. While she never panics, she does, on occasion, tend to err on the side of caution. This, apparently, was one of those times.

As it turned out, our regular pediatrician, Dr. Emory Baker, was not on call that night. Patsy spoke to his partner. After a few minutes of conversation, this doctor, who had not examined Michele recently, made a telephone diagnosis. It was the old "take two aspirins and call me in the morning" suggestion.

The doctor told Patsy to turn on a hot shower and let Michele breath the steam — that should do it, he said. It was a pattern we were to discover was routine with doctors who tend to see mostly well babies. To these doctors, many mothers are hysterical, many mothers over react to symptoms of stress in their children. While a few may do that, it's not always the case.

Patsy said, "I'm a nurse, doctor. This is not simple congestion. Something is wrong."

The doctor agreed to meet Patsy at his office to take a look at Michele, right away. Partly, we think, he agreed to see Michele because Patsy told him she was a nurse. You shouldn't have to be a nurse or a doctor or a paramedic to get a doctor's serious attention, but in the medical profession, many times they do tend to listen to you a little more closely if you are. It seems that many doctors believe that if you don't have any medical training you are therefore a complete medical moron. This is a attitude which runs through much of the profession, from surgeons to paramedics. More of them should listen a little more closely to the the patient and to the family. After all, who knows more about a child than the child's parent?

And a well informed parent, who is not kept in the dark by a sanctimonious M.D., can be the doctor's most valuable diagnostic resource. Always insist that your child's doctor make you a partner in your child's health care. If they resist doing that, find another doctor — fast.

As I stayed home with a suddenly very serious, very concerned big sister, Patsy drove off into the rainy night with our sick baby girl. While both Charlie and I were worried that Michele might have suffered a freak injury, neither of us were at all prepared for what lay ahead for Michele and for our family.

As Michele lay on the examining table, you could see a swelling in the area of her right kidney. The doctor asked how long it had been there. I had to admit that I had never seen it before. I bathed her, I dressed her each day and somehow I had missed this big lump in her tummy. How could I possibly have missed something like that? It was huge.

Perhaps it was because I was working evenings and two nights a week the baby sitter bathed the girls. My guilt had already begun to develop.

The doctor tried to hide his concern, but he did say that he felt we should take Michele directly to Childrens Hospital.

"That mass, whatever it is, should be evaluated as soon as possible, Mrs. Nolan," he said, trying hard not to alarm me.

I looked at him and said, "It's a Wilm's tumor."

It was a flat statement of fact, not a question.

He said, "There is no way to know that at this point, Mrs. Nolan. It could be many things. We have no way to know until we do a few tests."

"I know it could be many things, but I also know that it's a Wilm's," I said flatly.

Whether I really knew for sure it was a Wilm's tumor, or whether it was just some scary memory I had dredged up from nurses training, I will never know. I do know that I was suddenly scared nearly to death. I was shaking so much I could hardly drive back home. I knew in my heart, as I drove tearfully through the rain, that my three year old baby girl had cancer. Cancer of her right kidney.

The tumor turned out to be the size of a grapefruit, but these tumors grow at an alarming rate. The doctors later estimated that it had only started to grow a couple of weeks before the fall.

In falling, she had bruised the tumor and it had been bleeding into its capsule which in turn had caused an increase in pressure. The pressure was causing the pain that alerted us to the presence of the tumor. The fall, it turned out, had been a very good thing. Without the fall, it might have been days or even weeks before we learned of the tumor's existence.

When Patsy walked through the door holding Michele, she was as white as a sheet. She had the face of a woman looking death in the eye. My heart almost stopped. I had never seen that look on her face before, even when my dad was dying. This rainy night in Los Angeles, the look on my wife's face scared me to the very core of my being. Even before she spoke to me, I had never before experienced such a desperate feeling of fear and dread as I did that night when Pats walked through the door, carrying Michele.

"What's the matter?" I asked, not actually wanting to be told.

"We have to take Michele to the hospital."

"Tonight? In the morning? When?" I asked, completely stunned by this sudden, frightening news and still reeling from the look on Patsy's face.

"Tonight! Right now. She has something on her right kidney. The doctor's already called ahead.They're waiting for us at Childrens, honey."

"What's wrong with her?"

"The doctor doesn't know for sure. He wants the hospital to run some tests."

"Tonight?"

"Yes, right now. I'm going to call Sandy and ask her to keep Teresa," she said, now handing me a very lethargic, very tiny, and very still Michele.

Patsy never told me, until we started to write this book, that she had known that night that Michele had kidney cancer. She had tried to protect me from the horrible panic which she was experiencing.

As with most things in life, a little knowledge can be a terrible thing. Patsy's medical training had served us well through the struggle to save my dad and other times, but now with Michele, it would sometimes be the source of Patsy's increased anguish. Patsy simply knew too much.

There she was, on this first night, trying to insulate me from that terror by keeping from me what she already knew — it was very bad news about Michele and Michele's right kidney.

While Patrick rocked Michele, I called our friends, Sandy and Alan Muir. Without explaining why, I asked Sandy if I could bring Teresa over to their house for a few hours. The Muirs had two daughters who were almost exactly the same ages as Teresa and Michele.

Sandy, of course, said, yes. She would be happy to watch Teresa.

We hurriedly dropped Teresa at the Muir house, only a few blocks away, and started out through the rain for Childrens Hospital.

Before we had turned the first corner, Michele threw up everything she had in her stomach. It went all over her and all over me. We were both complete messes. Since we were just a few minutes away, we returned home to change clothes.

At the hospital that night, we spent what seems now to have been an eternity in the emergency room, having x-rays and blood tests taken and watching every guy in a white coat stop to do his own poking and prodding of Michele abdomen.

Michele's blood pressure when she was admitted was 170/140, terribly high, especially for a three year old.

Things seemed to be so desperate that night. We were just a little short of completely losing control of ourselves. Dad's death, in his sixties, had been one thing. This was our three year old baby, for God's sake.

Finally, after several hours, she was admitted to her room in a surgical ward upstairs. A young doctor, wearing a white lab coat, took us out of Michele's room into the hallway. He told us that they suspected she may have a malignant tumor, called a Wilm's, growing on her right kidney.

"I'm sorry, but it looks like your daughter may have cancer."

I thought I was going to stop breathing. Cancer! My baby girl has cancer? How can that be? There must be some horrible mistake!

The young doctor said there would be more tests tomorrow, including a kidney function test and then they might know for sure.

There was nothing more to do tonight and so he suggested that we go home and try to get some sleep. The nurses, who were very sympathetic, reassured us that they would take good care of our little girl. They knew we were scared. They just didn't know how scared.

The truth is, not everyone who works with children who are faced with a life threatening illness really does know how scared the parents are, unless they have experienced it first hand. When you're confronted with the serious possibility that your child might die, it's much more chilling than looking death in the eye for yourself. It's actually a feeling of utter terror. It's a fear you can actually feel at the back of your skull, in your bones, and in your gut.

Patsy said later that, as a nurse, she had always felt deeply for the parents who lost a child, a child who had been in her care. However, after Michele's sickness, it took on a whole new perspective for her.

Even as a loving grandparent, family member or close friend, you really can't know — nor can you even truly begin to understand — what a parent is going through at a time like this, unless, of course, you've walked a few miles in those shoes yourself.

Patrick and I stayed at the hospital that night just long enough to get Michele settled in bed, kiss her good night, then slowly leave for home. I felt like I was abandoning her when we walked out the front door of Childrens Hospital that night. My heart was heavy as we walked through the rain to our car. We didn't speak.

We went to the Muir's to fetch Teresa. The Muirs didn't know what to do to help. Alan looked grim. Sandy just cried. At a time like this there is nothing anyone can do. Nothing, that is, but be there to do what might be asked of you.

Most people will say, "What can I do?"

The answer normally is: nothing. There's nothing you can do and nothing you can say. You just need to be there. Just be there for those who are scared and in pain.

Now it was our turn to be there for someone. We had to be there for Teresa. She was very deeply concerned about her little sister.

We tried to tell her that while it looked serious, we'd know more tomorrow. Maybe it wasn't going to be as bad as we thought. But Teresa was a very bright, sensitive child who remembered very well the recent loss of her granddaddy. She could tell, even at seven years of age, that we were facing yet another serious family crises here. Consequently, she was very scared for her sister, her mother, her dad, and for herself.

We took Teresa home, spent some time trying to comfort her fears, put her to bed and climbed into bed ourselves. It was after midnight, but sleep was out of the question, at least for a little while. We both felt like we were a hundred years old with a ton of bricks sitting on our chests.

As we lay there in bed that night, waiting for sleep to ease the pain, we talked about our fears. Mainly we talked about our fear that Michele might be as sick as they suspected — something that Pats already knew, but that I was still rejecting. We talked about our fear that we might not be able to afford the best care for her. Our deepest fear, of course, was that Michele might die. We had to be prepared for that. It certainly was a possibility. A possibility that had to be faced, sooner or later.

Pats said she didn't know if she could deal with Michele's death, if it happened. I knew she could, but I didn't know if I could survive the loss of my child so soon after the loss of my father. God, I was terrified that night.

As I look back on it now, I'm sure my dad's death had taken more of a toll on Patsy than any of us had really understood at the time. We were all so wrapped up in our own grief, we hadn't taken a very close look at each other. She had loved my dad so very much, but had been forced to watch him slip from us, one horrible inch at a time. She had been there with him for so many nights in a row, without a break.

There, all alone with him in the middle of the night, she had watched my father painfully losing his courageous fight for life. It had taken a big toll on my partner.

Patsy said she just didn't think she could deal with another trauma like that, so soon after going through what she had gone through with Dad's illness. Dad had died just eighteen months ago.

Patsy was also going through what every Mother who has a baby with a serious illness — particularly a disease like cancer — goes through. She was sure that she was somehow to blame. Something the baby had inherited from her, something she had allowed the baby to come in contact with, something she had done — or had not done, had to be the cause of her child's illness. It's a normal reaction.

Guilt, particularly false guilt like this, can be a real killer. I'm sad to say that I didn't deal with Pats' feelings of guilt very well.

In truth, I don't think I really understood those feelings very well when I was thirty years old, either. I would later came to have a much better feel for that view, but I should have been more sensitive to those motherly feelings of guilt that night. I could have, and should have, provided more support for her and should have tried to do something to relieve those feelings of guilt. Patsy was suffering a great deal, mostly in silence.

Instead of asking for support, she tried to shield me from worrying too much about Michele. That night, Patsy tried to comfort me. She told me that Michele was going to be fine. She told me that cancer wasn't a death sentence — it was just another problem to solve and she said we would solve it together. Inside, of course, she was scared to death. We both were.

We both knew, instinctively, that we had to help each other if we were going to survive this and if we were going to help Michele in her battle with cancer. The only way we would get through the terrible days ahead would be if we were there to help each other.

It may be difficult to believe, but that night, as we lay there in the dark, I loved Patsy more than I had ever loved her before in my life. My heart was breaking because I knew she was hurting and I couldn't take away any of the pain. I knew she was thinking the same thing about me.

We finally drifted into sleep, crying, holding hands.

As I said earlier, I worked part time in the intensive care ward of a hospital near our home. Because I worked Friday, Saturday and Sunday nights, I had to call and tell them not to expect me any time in the near future.

The next morning Patrick and I went to Childrens Hospital and then he went on to work. I think problems like these seem easier on fathers than mothers, sometimes, because they are able to forget it for a while during their working hours. There were to be more tests and conferences with the doctors and discussions about what course of action to take. I knew that within a day or two we would be taking Michele to surgery.

This morning, after an entire evening of poking and prodding, Michele now had a hand-lettered sign over her bed that said, "Do Not Palpate Abdomen".

We did have a steady stream of young doctors in training who would stop by her bed, read her chart, touch her head, take her pulse and move on, wordlessly. It was going to be a long day and this parade of grim faced, white coated medicine men were not making it any easier on me. Few of them spoke. They just stopped, added to their medical knowledge and moved on to another child.

Someone who was thinking like a person had placed rocking chairs in every room at Childrens Hospital. Throughout the early morning hours, I sat with Michele on my lap and softly rocked her in that wonderful chair. Occasionally she would stir and ask for something to drink. I had to tell her that she was not allowed to have anything to drink. I told her she was getting all her drinks through the IV. Because of the tests that were scheduled, she couldn't have anything by mouth — NPO in hospital lingo. I did manage to get a wet wash cloth so she could moisten her mouth.

Around nine that morning an orderly came to take Michele to x-ray for an IVP, an x-ray of her kidneys, taken after a special dye has been injected into her veins. I went downstairs with her, staying at her side as they put a needle into her tiny foot. She didn't cry, she didn't fuss, she just lay there, looking back at me with those huge, blue eyes.

I said a tearful goodbye to Patsy at the hospital, after I had wished Michele a good morning, telling her how much her father loved her.

By the time I got to the KHJ-TV studios on Melrose Avenue, the word had already spread throughout the building that Michele was sick. During the past evening I had called Walt Baker from the hospital to tell him I might not be available to work the next day. Walt's a very old and very dear friend of ours. I really just needed to talk to him more than anything else. I was scared to death and Walter can be a tower of strength. He's been there for me more than once.

Walt had told my boss, Milt Hoffman, that I might not be in, that our daughter was gravely ill and that we'd know more this morning. Within five minutes everyone else in the building knew that Michele was hospitalized. They also knew that it was probably very serious. Their outpouring of concern meant a great deal to me that morning. I'll never forget how everyone in the building wore his heart on his sleeve that day.

Milt was waiting at the top of the stairs when I came up. He looked like he'd just been given a death sentence. This tough, hard nosed television veteran was hurting.

"What's happening?," he asked.

"She's in the hospital."

"I KNOW that," he interrupted. "What else do you know?"

Milt was an intense sort of guy — always in control, but this morning he seemed to be quite upset by the news of our daughter's illness. I had seen him angry a lot of times (usually with me). I had seen him upset, tired, stressed, and in lots of situations that one might describe as filled with pressure, but I'd never seen this particular look on his face. As a matter of fact, I can't remember seeing that expression on anyone's face — before or since.

"She has a tumor on her kidney, Milt. It looks like it might be cancer," I said, as gently as I could.

Cancer is a word that strikes terror into the hearts of most of us — Milt Hoffman is definitely one of those people. He looked like he was going to be sick to his stomach. I really felt very sorry for him. The news of

51

our little one having cancer was ripping a hole in this tough "I can handle anything" Hollywood producer.

He put his arm around me. Milt's a lot like me in that way, always touching people when he talks to them. I have a great picture of Milt with his hand on my shoulder as we stood on the floor of the studio, during one of our shows. I love that picture. I'll always believe that Milt Hoffman really liked me. Although he never told me so, I'll always just be happy thinking that he did.

"What the hell can we do, kid? Is there anything anyone can do?"

"Nothing that I know of, Milt. There doing more tests this morning. We should know more by noon," I said.

"When you know, I want to know. OK?"

"Sure. And thanks, Milt."

"You sure you should be here? Maybe you should be with your wife at the hospital."

"Milt, we've got a show to do and things are calm there, right now, at least. I need to be busy, but I'll let you know what she says when Pats calls."

"Okay. Be sure you do."

He gave my shoulder a hug and walked down the hall. This guy was a prince. I'll never forget his show of concern and his love that morning.

Milt, if you read this book, I just want to say, "Thanks, Pal." Your reaching out to me that morning, with your genuine feelings of love and genuine concern, meant more to me than I can tell you — even now — so just know that I have never forgotten that moment with you at the top of the stairs at old KHJ-TV.

Dr. Emory Baker, Michele's regular pediatrician came in to see me about 10:30.

"Mrs. Nolan," he said softly, but professionally, "There is a large tumor on your daughter's right kidney. We won't know until after the surgery what kind it is, or for that matter whether or not it is malignant. The most common tumor on children of Michele's age is a Wilm's tumor, however. Wilm's are, as you know, malignant growths."

I caught my breath. I had known, in my heart, since last night at the doctor's office that Michele had a Wilm's tumor, but having been told, if even unofficially, made my legs weak and my throat dry. Michele has cancer. How would I ever be able to tell Patrick?

"I have contacted a pediatric surgeon, Dr. Morton Woolley. He's the best in town. He will be here to see you sometime this afternoon," Dr. Baker said as he touched my arm before leaving the room.

There are times in our lives that we revert to being children, and for me this was such a time. I went to the phone and called my mother in Boulder City, Nevada.

"Mama, Michele is in the hospital and they are going to operate on her. They think she has cancer. Can you come down?"

Here I was, a married woman of thirty-three, with a loving husband and two children, but I didn't call my husband, I called my mother. Mothers are supposed to make things better. I wanted my mama to take this all away. That way Patrick wouldn't have to suffer with this terrible burden. I would never have to say to him that Michele had cancer, if mom would just make it all go away.

Mama, of course, couldn't make it all go away, but she told me that she's be at our house that evening. She'd call my brother, Barry Whalen, who also lived in Los Angeles, and have him meet her at the airport. Barry would bring her to the house.

After I hung up, I called Patrick at the studio. I knew all along that I would have to call him, but I hated doing it.

"The doctor was just here, honey. The tumor is attached to the right kidney and they think it's a Wilm's tumor," I said through my tears.

"What the hell does that mean?"

"It means," I said, "that it's probably cancer. The surgeon will be in this afternoon to talk about taking it out. She's been sleeping since she came back from x-ray. She doesn't seem to be in as much pain today."

We went on the air with "Tempo" at noon every day — live. I was the on-air producer, orchestrating all the elements that went into the show as we broadcast it. It was my decision when a guest was introduced, when to break for a commercial, when to break for news, when to take calls from the audience, where to put a newsmaker call, and when to say goodbye to a guest or when — and sometimes, how — to end a segment. I always said it was like leading a big jazz band. If I did my job right, everyone else looked good. If I was missing the beat, we all looked like flaming idiots.

Normally, I was very good at my job and I loved doing it. But, not this day. Today I hated being here in this windowless room with its forty odd monitors and nervous people who didn't seem to know what to say to me. Some of them tried not to look at me.

On Friday, November 15, 1968, I wasn't even in L.A., much less the studios of KHJ. I was somewhere out in space, dying. I could barely breath. As the show began, I began to get more and more frightened, more and more anxious. It was a terrible feeling of helplessness.

Every minute the anxiety seemed to get worse. I missed breaks, I forgot to give the right cues to the talent. I let the show run over into the news. I wasn't, as musicians say, playing on the same page as the rest of the cast and crew. They were trying to help me, but I was causing the show to "crash and burn."

The pit of my stomach was churning. My nerves were shot and I was getting more upset by the minute. What, I thought to myself, was I doing in this cold control room? I belonged with Patsy. I belonged at the hospital with my partner and our sick child.

I grabbed the phone, dialed Walter's direct extension and said, "Walt, I've got to get the hell out of here. I'm sorry. I need to be at the hospital. Can you come down and finish the show for me?"

"Go. Don't wait for me. I'll be right down. They can fake it 'til I get there," he said as he hung up.

I gave a few last minute instructions to a grim faced crew who all wished me good luck, then I whispered a quick goodbye on the telex into the ears of my hosts who were on the air, busy with a guest, and ran out the back door of the studio to my parking space. The hospital was only about three miles down Sunset Boulevard. I drove there through my tears.

I had been sitting, holding Michele, in the rocking chair for several hours. It seemed to me that she grew smaller and smaller as the hours passed. Logically, of course, I know that it wasn't possible for her to grow smaller in my arms, but that's what I felt was happening as we rocked away the afternoon. I felt she was just slipping away from me, getting smaller and smaller. Soon, I was sure, she would just be gone.

When I walked into Michele's room that afternoon, Patsy was sitting in a big white rocking chair, holding Michele across her lap. Michele looked drugged and I guess she was, to some extent. She had had a rough night and a long day of x-rays and blood tests and kidney function tests. She'd been poked, stuck, thumped, turned, carried, prodded, examined, and reexamined. She was completely worn out.

She was also one very sick little girl.

Even today I still can vividly see that tragic scene as I walked through the door into Michele's hospital room. Just the thought of that tragic scene still makes me cry. It is one of the worst memories of my whole life. I felt so desperate. The white fear of what was happening to my little baby and the pain that my partner was feeling were almost too much for me to bear. That scene, with them sitting there in that rocking chair, has been a haunting memory for me ever since that terrible day.

We knew by now that tomorrow morning Morton Woolley, M.D. was going to operate on our three year old daughter and remove a huge kidney tumor. We didn't know — and they didn't know — how much more was involved or what else they might find during the operation. Those terrible things we didn't know, but could certainly imagine, were driving us both crazy. The fact that Michele had cancer was one thing. Not knowing what it actually might mean after tomorrow's surgery was even more frightening.

Late that afternoon, I met Morton Woolley for the first time. He came into the room and walked over to the other side of Michele's bed.

"Mr. and Mrs. Nolan, I'm Doctor Woolley."

He was wearing a shiny silk suit and a silk tie with a big, ugly tie clasp right across the middle of it. The clasp was longer than the width of his tie. It was an expensive, suit, complete with a shirt that had a collar about two sizes bigger than his neck. He looked like a guy who was wearing clothes belonging to someone else. He might be able to afford that suit, I remember thinking, but he sure as hell didn't wear it very well.

"Jeez," I also thought to myself, "I sure hope this guy can operate better than he dresses."

Woolley was cool and very detached — distant, aloof and superior. Patsy had told me that Dr. Baker said Woolley was the finest pediatric surgeon in L.A. He was the best there was and, of course, we wanted the very best for Michele. Everyone wants the very best for his child.

Woolley said that the operation would be at seven the following day and that it would probably take four or five hours.

He said that the anesthesiologist would also be by this evening and then he asked the question that most doctors ask, "Do you have any questions?"

And we did what all scared-to-death parents do when they're faced with that awful question. We just shook our heads and muttered, no. We didn't know what to ask.

It has taken me years to sort through my feelings about this unfortunate, but oft asked question. It's a question I will never again allow any expert, particularly a medical expert, to ask me without challenging it, immediately.

At a time like this, in the first few hours after learning that your child has cancer, you are so very vulnerable, so defenseless. You are absolutely scared to death. Absolutely terrified to the roots of your teeth. At a time like this, you find yourself grasping at straws of hope wherever you think you might find them.

In this situation especially, just before major surgery on a baby, one hesitates to ask the doctor anything. Partly, I believe, out of an unconscious fear that if you ask a question the doctor doesn't have an answer for, it will upset him (or her). The last thing in the world you want at a time like this, is for the anointed savior of your child to become upset at anything, but you particularly do not want him to become upset with you. Walking on eggs while wearing golf shoes would be easier then asking a question which might upset your child's surgeon.

At a terrible time like this, you are standing there with a knot in your stomach and your heart in your throat. You feel so deeply grateful that this talented, gifted, highly educated individual has agreed to reach down from his lofty position and save the life of your child. You are so grateful to him that you almost genuflect in his presence. You almost certainly always lower your eyes in a clear gesture of subservience. With total command of the situation, the doctor calls all the shots.

Morton Woolley certainly had this technique down cold. He was a master at projecting a near God-like attitude. Terrified parents didn't ask this guy anything.

"I'll see you, tomorrow, after the surgery," he said.

Little did we know at that moment, the night before the surgery, just how hollow, that simple promise would turn out to be.

He said good night and walked out of Michele's room in his shiny, silk suit with the bad tie clip.

That night, we left at the end of visiting hours, picking up Teresa from the Muir's where she had gone after school.

Teresa asked, "Momma, is Michele in a pink hospital?"

I told her that I thought it was grey.

She said, "That's good. Because Granddaddy died in a pink hospital and I don't want Michele to die."

You can never be sure what goes on inside a child's mind.

The three of us drove home, ate a little dinner and went to bed.

When Patrick and I were in bed, one of us, I really don't remember which one of us, asked, "Will you please make love with me? I need to be as close to you as I can."

For some reason it was very important to both Patrick and me that we make love that night. We didn't need to have sex. We both just needed to be as close to each other as we possibly could be, at that moment. And we were.

As far as I can remember, before we wrote this book, neither one of us had ever shared that very personal moment with anyone. We have elected to share that moment with you here because we want the mothers and fathers who may find themselves in the same situation — and who may read this book — to know that it's okay to feel the need to be that close to your partner. It's very important to feel that you must be that close. If you just go to sleep, you may cause your mate to feel that you're turning away in some way. Don't turn away. You need each other more than at any other time in your marriage. Be there for each other. It's okay.

At a deep, emotional and highly charged crisis like this, the importance to renew your absolute, total commitment to each other can not be expressed strongly enough here. There's just no better way to make that commitment known than to make love to your partner.

On Saturday morning, November 16, 1968, we arrived at the hospital about seven-thirty.

The first thing Michele asked for was a drink of water.

"I'm sorry, honey, but you can't have anything to drink or anything to eat until after the operation."

"Why not, Daddy?"

"Because they don't want you to be sick to your stomach during the surgery. That would be very bad."

"I won't be sick. I promise," she pleaded.

My heart was breaking. We had told her that she was going to go to sleep and that they were going to operate to remove that painful lump in her tummy. A lump that was by now, after all the poking and prodding, very sore. We had told her not to be frightened, that everyone here loved her and wanted her to get well.

She seemed, intuitively, to understand how sick she was, even though she was only three years old. Walt Baker's wife, Sally, said that Michele was three, going on thirty-three. I think Sally hit the nail right on the head.

"Listen," I said, "when you wake up, if you still want one, you can have a drink of water."

Of course, I never thought for a moment that she would still want a drink of water after surgery.

"Promise?"

"Promise! If you still want a drink when you wake up, you can have one," I told her.

That turned out to be a real dumb promise to make, but at a moment like this, just before they take your child off to surgery, maybe never to return, you will promise anything. But try not to promise anything you can't deliver, like I did that morning. You may live to regret it. I did.

Before we knew it, it was time for them to take her away. We walked all the way to the operating suite with her. She was pretty groggy from the pre-op shots, but she was awake and she still wanted a drink. While she didn't get one, she didn't get upset about it, either. She just made Patrick promise, one more time before she was taken through those awful double doors, that he would get her a drink as soon as she woke up. He, of course, again promised her that he would.

The orderlies and a nurse wheeled Michele's bed through the doors at nine-thirty that morning. Patrick and I both told her that we loved her. In a blink, she was out of sight. That was a very tough moment. But tougher moments waited in the shadows.

It was Saturday morning. Our good friend, Mildred Hudec was up from Yucaipa to be with us. She's a wonderful friend. My mom was up from Indio. I knew, so soon after dad's terrible struggle, that this continued to be a tough time for mom. I hated adding to her grief.

Patsy's mom had flown in from Boulder City the night before and was at our home with Teresa. Lillian Whalen would stay with us as long as we needed her.

It was good to have all of them and their love around us there, as we waited through the operation, but, in truth, Patsy and I were really pretty much alone that day. We were there alone with each other while the beautiful issue of our love was upstairs on a small, cold table, under a bright white light. We were just going to have to hold on to each other and wait out the time it would take. Time went by very slowly that day.

At 1:50 in the afternoon, after four and a half long hours, a nurse came to the waiting room and said, "They're just closing now. Dr. Woolley should be down to see you in about fifteen minutes. Please stay right here so he will know where to find you."

We thanked her and watched the elevator doors.

Fifteen minutes, twenty minutes, thirty minutes went by with no sign of Morton Woolley.

Patsy and I both knew that something terrible must have gone wrong at the last minute. What other explanation could there possible be for his delay?

Mildred Hudec's face was filled with dread. She knew it meant something very bad, too. My mom was holding it together, but she was starting to become a little frightened as well.

Woolley should have finished by now and been down to tell us what he had found and what he had done to our baby. The nurse said they were finished. The minutes ticked by and still he didn't show. That could only mean that there was a problem. I can't tell you how this waiting — after being told they were finished and closing — deepened our fears.

Patsy, having been a scrub nurse during a lot of operations, knew that sometimes something can go sour at the last second. After forty-five minutes, we just knew it meant that the worst had happened. Michele was either dead or in some terrible additional jeopardy.

I just couldn't wait any longer. I was going nuts. I told Patsy to stay in the waiting room, just in case Woolley did show up. I went up to Michele's floor to asked the nurse to call into the OR and find out what the problem was with Michele. I was in a state of semi-panic. I had to know what the hell had gone wrong. After six hours of surgery, I had to know if we'd lost Michele.

The nurse called the operating room supervisor. Michele wasn't in the operating room.

"Then where the hell is she?" I demanded.

My semi-panic moved to near panic. Where the hell was Michele?

What had happened? What was going on here?

The nurse, sensing my severe anxiety, called the recovery room. As she listened to the person on the other end of the phone, her face relaxed. She smiled.

"Everything's fine, Mr. Nolan. Michele's in recovery. She's been there for more than half an hour and she's doing just great. She'll be in ICU in about another thirty minutes," she told me.

"Where is Dr. Woolley? What did they find? What did they do?" I asked.

"I'm sure he's on his way to see you and your wife. He may be in the waiting room with your wife, right now," she said, trying to reassure me with the party line.

She was trying to calm me down, but it wasn't working. I was starting to get very agitated.

"She's fine. She's in recovery. Has Woolley been here?" I asked as I got off the elevator. As a group, Patsy and the others just shook their heads.

"I've got to find a phone."

I asked the hospital operator if she would page Dr. Morton Woolley.

Now, I was becoming really upset. We needed to find out what had happened during those terrifying five hours. Was it really cancer? Did he get it all out? What were the chances that she might die? We were loaded with unanswered questions and we needed some answers. What the hell had happened to Woolley?

"I'm sorry, Dr. Woolley has checked out of the hospital," the operator calmly informed me.

"Can't be," I said.

"I'm sorry, but he's left for the day, sir," she assured me.

"Are you absolutely positive?" I demanded, in total disbelief of what she was telling me.

"Yes, I am, sir. Dr. Woolley has left for the day. You'll have to reach him through his office tomorrow. I'm sorry."

Sorry? I was becoming a complete basket case by now. What the hell was going on here? Why didn't Woolley come down to talk to us? My stress level, already near critical mass, was rising.

This time Patsy and I both went back to the nurses station, leaving Mom and Mildred in the waiting room, just in case the operator was in error and Woolley was just slow changing back into that expensive silk suit.

"If he shows up here, sit on him. Don't let him leave for any reason," I told Mildred and mom as the elevator doors closed, confident that I had assigned the right job to the right two people.

When Pats and I got upstairs, the nurse could tell from my expression that we had not found Woolley.

"Can you tell me anything about Michele's operation?" I asked.

"No, I'm sorry I can't. I have no information. Michele's not here, yet so I don't have her chart. She's still in recovery. I can't believe Dr. Woolley hasn't come to talk to you."

"Believe it," Patsy said, coldly. "He left the hospital."

"Maybe he got tied up with another patient," the nurse suggested.

"And maybe not. We haven't seen him since last night. The hospital operator told us that he checked out of the hospital right after the surgery," Patsy said with that cutting edge in her voice that means she's had had all of this she is going to tolerate. Over the years, the kids and I learned, the hard way, about that tone in her voice.

The nurse seemed to clearly understand that Patsy wasn't going to allow any more double talk.

"And he didn't come talk to you?"

Patsy couldn't believe that she was hearing the same question, again.

"He left, damn it! He left the hospital without talking to us. What kind of a jerk is this guy?"

"Oh, my God. I'm really sorry. Let me try to find the surgeon who assisted him. Give me a minute. I'm sure he's still here," she said.

The nurse was obviously upset that Woolley hadn't come right down from surgery to see us. She was in total disbelief when we told her that he had just walked out the door and gone home, without bothering to see us after major surgery on a toddler.

The nurse made three or four calls before she located Dr. Abraham Mares, a young, senior surgical resident — Childrens is, after all, a teaching hospital — who had assisted in Michele's surgery. Dr. Mares was doing rounds on the sixth floor. We raced up the stairs, not waiting for an elevator, not waiting for Dr. Mares to find us. We would find him.

Dr. Mares was with a small child in a room on the sixth floor when we found him. He was deeply embarrassed that Woolley had not been to see us. In fact, he didn't believe us.

"If he talked to anyone, he talked to total strangers," I said. "We haven't seen him, please believe me. Now, tell us about Michele and the surgery, please."

He told us that the surgery had gone well, that Michele had tolerated the procedure very well. It had been a very large Wilm's, involving the entire right kidney, which had also been removed,

"There was just nothing left of the right kidney. The tumor had almost completely encapsulated it," he explained.

He went on to tell us that they had also removed part of her right adrenal gland and her appendix. He told us that in a few minutes he was going to head down to ICU to check on her condition. We told him we would meet him there. For the moment, I put Woolley out of my mind. I just wanted to see Michele, alive.

With tubes in both arms, in her chest, up her nose and down her throat into her stomach and into her bladder, Michele was a frightening sight for a scared young father and mother to behold.

Her tummy was painted that bright orange from the antiseptic. There was a light dressing over an enormous wound that had a drain tube running out of it. Fragile and delicate, she looked like she had lost half — or more — of her body weight. Michele looked for all the world like a lab experiment.

I leaned down and kissed her as gently as I could. She opened her eyes and looked at me from deep within two very sunken eye sockets. Those huge blue eyes were looking up at me from the back of her skull.

"Where's my drink of water?" she wanted to know.

My eyes filled with tears. I knew she couldn't have even a sip of water, but I also knew that Patrick had promised her one. And at our house, a promise is a promise, period. He was now between a big rock and a very hard spot. I knew he'd have to break that promise because there was no way anyone wanted that frail little body, with its huge incision, to undergo the strain of vomiting.

Patrick knelt on the floor beside her bed, begging her to let him off the hook on this one.

"I'm sorry, honey, you just can't have a drink just yet. It might make you throw up and we can't let you do that. It might do some damage to your operation," I told her as I softly touched her head.

Patrick was the one who was dying.

"I won't throw up. I promise. But I'm very thirsty," she pleaded as her eyes filled with tears.

I leaned down to tried, again, to bail Patrick out of the tough spot he's gotten himself into.

"Michele, the doctor doesn't want you to have anything to drink. It's not Daddy's fault. It's doctor's orders. It might make you sick."

She started to cry a little, but she was only able to produce one huge tear. I wiped it away and squeezed Patrick's shoulder. I knew this was killing him. I also knew that her anesthesiologist had been a genius. He had brought her out so carefully that she wasn't the least bit nauseated. His work had been a work of art. To hell with Woolley's skills, the anesthesiologist was the magician here and we didn't want to spoil what he'd accomplished with something as silly as a drink of water, promised by her father, or not.

At that moment an orderly, who had been assigned to care for her gently wiped Michele's face with a cool, damp cloth. This guy had the enormous hands with the fingers of a football linebacker, but the touch of an angel.

He put his big face down near her ear and almost whispered, "I'll get you a lemon stick in just a few minutes. You'll like that. It will be even better than a drink. Now, let's not cry and get tears all over your bandages. Okay?"

That guy saved my life.

"Okay," Michele sighed, resigned now to the fact that she wasn't going to get any water. At least not right now.

All through the next two years — and even now, as an adult — Michele developed a most pragmatic outlook on life. If there was something that arguing and fussing over wasn't going to change, she just keep quiet and did what was asked of her.

If, however, there was an opportunity to influence or change someone's mind, or point out that an injustice was about to be perpetrated, she was totally ruthless. She was also very good at figuring out how to have some small measure of control over her situation, even at that tender age.

For instance, later she would make a deal with the lab technicians when it came to the daily — sometimes twice daily — blood tests. While there was no way out of it, she could do something to make it less painful and less frightening.

Although I was only three years old at the time, I have a clear memory of the technic I used to remain — if only a tiny bit — in control.

I didn't want them to stab the end of my finger with that sharp, little blade that they used to use to draw blood for a blood smear. That thing was just like the point of an exacto blade and it hurt like mad. Over the years I have had hundreds of those little blood smears taken during the surgeries, the radiation treatments and the subsequent chemotherapy treatments. There wasn't one that didn't hurt and hurt badly. I hated that "finger stick," as they call it, worse than just about anything else. But I was also totally aware that they were going to do it, no matter how much I fussed. Knowing that it was going to happen anyway, I used this opportunity to make a deal with the lab technicians.

"If I get to pick the finger, I won't cry," I assured them.

It wasn't that this was going to stop it from hurting. It was going to hurt, no matter what deal I made. There was no way for anyone else to tell which one was sore by looking at my fingers. But sometimes they picked the same finger that had been stabbed the day before or even that same day. In a few hours the skin was completely back to normal, but the damage to those tender nerves below the surface took days to heal. While sticking a "new" finger still kills, stabbing that thing into the tip of a finger that had recently been stabbed and was already very sore, was pure murder. I knew, even at that young age, that if I could pick the finger, I could pick the one that had healed the most. It may have been only a small thing to think about — at a time when a lot of real scary things are going on around you, but you'd be surprised how much difference a little something like that can make in the mind of a three year old. It gave me a tiny amount of control over my life at a time when I didn't have any.

For me, that first couple of hours after the surgery became a blur.

Patrick's mom, Charlotte, and my dear friend, Mildred Hudec, had to be thanked, and sent home, with our love. It had been a hard day for both of these wonderful women. It was a long, lonely drive home for them, I'm sure, but I was so very grateful that they had been there with us that day. Even though there was nothing either of them could do for us. Just their being there that day still means a lot to me.

Patrick went home to tell Mama and Teresa that Michele was through the surgery and that she was doing as well as we could expect. I knew that Mama would then call Dad in Boulder City, as well as my brothers and my sister, and let them know what had happened, so far.

Patrick and I were both exhausted from the strain and from the fear. It takes a tremendous amount of physical energy to be that scared.

Patrick came back to the hospital before dinner and took me home. Michele was in the very capable hands of a staff of loving, caring and very competent doctors and nurses who worked in the ICU at Childrens Hospital in Los Angeles. Even though I knew she would get the best of care during the night, it was still very hard to leave her there and go home that first night.

Before we turned in for the night, I called to check on her. She was doing fine. She was sleeping peacefully. Her vital signs were stable.

We could have stayed at the hospital, I suppose, but it seemed so important for all of us that we be with Teresa as well as Michele. We went home to say that life must go on, as normally as possible.

The next day was Sunday morning and we arrived at the hospital at a very early hour. We went into the cafeteria to get a cup of coffee before going upstairs to Michele and who should we find there, but the phantom of the surgery, Morton Woolley, M.D.

He didn't recognize us, of course. He had only met us once, on Friday evening before the surgery. We introduced ourselves to him.

Yes, of course, he said, the Nolans. No, he hadn't seen Michele, yet. He was just on his way up to check on her.

"We'd like to talk to you, after you've seen her. Shall we follow you?"

No, he had said. He did have a few other patients to see. But after he saw Michele he would find us.

"Where do you want us to wait?" I asked.

He suggested we wait right there in the cafeteria for a few minutes. He assured us both that he would come down after visiting Michele and checking her chart and give us the latest on her condition. We told him we'd stay right there, waiting.

At that time, both Patsy and I were still so scared of those guys in white coats that neither one of us had the nerve to ask Woolley about yesterday and his disappearing act after the surgery.

It seems, on reflection, that at a time like this, you're so frightened that you believe if you confront the doctor, he will, somehow, give your child less than the best care. You fear that he'll take out any hostility you may engender with even the slightest confrontation, on your child. Subsequently, you tend to treat your child's physicians as though they were completely above any reproach. It may be an unreasonable thing to believe, but it's there, nonetheless. Or, I should say, it once was there with me, but no more.

We waited there in the hospital cafeteria for two hours, not seeing Michele while we once again worried ourselves half sick over what might be the cause of Woolley's failure to return. Of course, we rationalized, he must have become involved with another child, that was the reason he was delayed. It was a very long two hours.

Finally, I decided I wasn't going to wait any longer. I headed for the phone. The hospital operator told me the same thing she had told me the day before, "I'm sorry, Dr. Woolley has checked out of the hospital for the day."

That SOB. He'd done it to us again!

As he walked in, the doctor, routinely, asked,
"How are you this morning, Michele?"
...this fragile little three year old baby, suffering the pain
and trauma of the first day after major surgery,
looked up with those big,dark, sunken eyes and said,
"Fine, thank you."

Chapter Four

"Fine, Thank you!"

I couldn't believe what I was told. That guy Woolley had pulled his disappearing act again, without talking to us. He just walked out, leaving us cooling our heels for worry-filled minute after worry-filled minute. Patsy and I just shook our heads collectively and went upstairs to see Michele.

At the time, neither of us fully realized the deep degree of anxiety and the feelings of raw, shear, white terror that this thoughtless, inconsiderate man had been responsible for generating in each of us with his two acts of unkindness.

As it turned out, I had been trying to shield my feelings of dread and the full impact those feelings were having on my stomach lining from Patsy as she was trying to keep me from seeing just how terrified she was as a result of having been left for hours, expecting the worst and knowing, as more and more time passed without any contact, that the news was going to be the worst possible news.

Woolley's abandonment of us — twice — without a thought to what that would do to raise the level of terror and anxiety in both of us, is without a doubt, the cruelest thing anyone has ever done to me.

As the years since those two awful days have passed, I began to think of it as a perverted, arrogant sort of cruelty. The absence of even the slightest degree of sensitivity makes me question this man's very humanity.

One thing I know for sure, Morton Woolley didn't go into the field of medicine to ease pain, reduce suffering or save lives.

Whatever happened to those wonderful days when the doctor was the most respected man in the community? A gentle, kind man who lived in a nice house, but not the biggest in town.Whatever happened to the days when our family doctor was a man who came to our house and drove a Buick?

Over twenty-five years have passed since those terrible days in Los Angeles, but the sheer anguish generated by Woolley's callous actions still returns to haunt me whenever I remember the insensitive manner of that man. Woolley, if you're reading this, I still haven't forgiven you and what you did to us. And I will never forget it.

However, back then, on her first post operative day after major surgery for kidney cancer, Michele, and not our own feelings and fears, was our most important concern. Dealing effectively with Woolley and his horrible methods of terrorizing two scared young parents of a child with cancer would just have to wait until another day.

When we got upstairs to ICU and to Michele, we could see a marked improvement from the evening before. The fluids they were pumping into her veins, and her own internal desire to live, had started the healing process. She was still a very sick little girl who had just survived a major abdominal operation for cancer, but she was looking a little better. I guess it would have been tough for her to have looked any worse than she did the day before, just hours after surgery.

A few minutes after we arrived at her bedside, one of the hospital's young resident physicians — a doctor still in training — gently approached her bed.

"How are you this morning, Michele?" he asked somewhat routinely, tenderly touching her face.

Her response to that simple, standard question proved to be our family's rallying cry for the next twenty-five years.

Here she was, trapped in the windowless maze of ICU, with vital fluids and healing medications running through plastic tubes into the veins in both of her frail arms and a heart monitor beeping away over her head. A drain from the huge incision in her orange painted abdomen dripped red liquid into a sump under the bed. A suction pump connected to her tube which had been inserted into her chest cavity through a puncture wound between two of her ribs, hissed as it evacuated air from the space around her lungs. There was a foley catheter in her bladder. She gagged on that awful nasogastric tube running up into her nose and down into her stomach, and she was in an oxygen tent which covered her and the whole gaggle of tubes, wires and gadgets.

With all of this happening to her, this fragile little three year old baby, with a fresh incision that ran from the middle of her back around her left side until it passed the right side to her belly button and suffering from all pain and trauma that is always associated with major surgery, she looked up with those big, dark, sunken eyes and replied to the doctor, "Fine, thank you."

Fine, thank you?

In a barely audible voice, here in this alien spaceship, she told this young doctor that she was just "Fine, thank you."

The full impact of her reply took a second or two. Then a wonderful expression came over the young physician's face as he smiled warmly at Patsy and me.

"Well, Michele," he said, touching her tiny arm, "we're going to see if we can't make you feel even better, sweetie."

I'm not sure, but I think I saw a tear in one corner of his eye as the young man turned to his morning's work, shaking his head in total disbelief.

Michele's incredibly naive response to a standard medical greeting had, under these circumstances, made a tremendous impression on this young doctor. It had, in fact, added an important lesson to his medical training. Here a tiny patient, who should have been completely overwhelmed by her

64

life threatening circumstances, her multiple discomforts and her imprisonment in this strange world of intensive care, was making a valiant attempt not to add to her doctor's concerns.

Here was a very special, and very unique, little human being who was making no demands, issuing no complaints. Nothing here was so bad that she needed to trouble anyone with it. This brave little kid was giving us all just another example of how she seemed to know, instinctively, that there were things which complaining about could alter and there were other things that would just have to be endured, without complaint — even without comment. It was a trait she had apparently inherited from one or both of her grandfathers.

The young resident told us more about what he had learned from reading her chart and from his conversations with Woolley. He told us what had been done in surgery, what they had found and what the future might hold. He was very forthcoming.

"We have every expectation that she can survive this disease," he optimistically told us.

"We're being more successful every day with Wilm's tumor. Our biggest fear, right now, aside from seeing that she recovers from the trauma of the surgery, is that her other kidney or her liver do not become affected. We'll want to begin radiation therapy and chemotherapy as soon as possible. Possibly as soon as tomorrow morning. This Wilm's stuff moves very, very fast, as you may know."

This bright young resident was developing a very fine bedside manner, unlike a lot of his colleagues. He was patient. He was thoughtful. And he was very sensitive to the vibrations, body language and small clues which he received from both his tiny patients and from their families. This guy actually listened. I'm sure he turned out to be a terrific physician. I wish one of us could remember his name.

Woolley had ordered a complete blood study to be done on Michele. That means drawing a big syringe of blood, as much as 20ccs, from her veins. That's a lot of blood from such a tiny body.

A young doctor by the name of Harvey Kershnar was assigned to follow Michele's case as she recovered from the operation. Dr. Kershnar had a nice touch.

"Michele," he said, "I have to take some blood from your arm. I want you to promise me that you'll hold as still as you can. Okay?"

"Is it going to hurt?" she asked. She'd had about all the pain she wanted at this point. Even a little more might be difficult to add to what she was already dealing with this morning.

We now watched as unteachable instincts took over for this young doctor. This is a part of a priceless, intuitive knowledge that only a few of the best physicians ever develop, even after years of practicing medicine. Here was a guy, still in his twenties, still learning medicine, who already knew a lot more about being a physician than doctors like Woolley would ever know in a lifetime. Dr. Kershnar had a wonderful bedside manner.

"Yes, Michele. It's going to hurt a little," he told her truthfully.

"Then I'm going to cry," she promised.

"You can cry, but I don't want you to move," he told her.

"I won't move, but I will cry," she promised him, rather sternly.

A nurse, much less sensitive to her patient than this young doctor, brought forth a child's arm board. It's a scary contraption used to strap a youngster's arm down so the patient can't pull away or fold their arm up when the needle gets close. It looks like a tool of medieval torture.

"You won't need that," Patrick told her.

She looked at the doctor for support. He only motioned to her to set it aside. The nurse looked skeptically at Patrick, wishing once again, that the parents would not interfere with how she did her job. After all, she must have thought, what did parents know?

"If she says she won't move, she won't move. That thing will just scare her," Patrick told the nurse, gently.

"I think we'll be just fine if you simply hold her arm steady, nurse," the doctor tactfully suggested.

The nurse, without completely accepting his decision, took a firm grip on Michele's pipe stem of an arm. Michele instantly started to cry.

"You told me you wouldn't cry until it hurt, Michele. I haven't done anything yet," the doctor said in a soothing tone, trying to gain her confidence and relax her.

"It does hurt!" Michele said emphatically.

Patrick looked down and saw that Michele's fingers were turning blue. This inflexible nurse had gripped Michele's arm so tightly that she was inflicting needless pain on her young patient.

"Here, let me do that," Patrick said, removing the nurses fingers from Michele's wrist and taking over.

The nurse glared at Patrick, "I'm sorry, you'll have to wait outside," she said, looking at the doctor, knowing he would overrule Patrick.

The doctor said nothing.

"I'm sorry, but we can't allow you to do that," the nurse again objected.

"Yes, you can," Patrick said. "We'll be just fine, nurse. I really do know what I'm doing and I really do know what needs to be done for my daughter."

"I think we'll be okay, nurse. Thank you," Dr. Kershnar said, acknowledging Patrick's perfectly correct appraisal of the situation.

Dr. Kershnar was willing to gently admonish this nurse in the presence of a couple of civilians because he recognized that what was important here was to deliver the best possible care, with the least possible additional trauma, to a fragile, gravely ill little patient. The nurse's personal feelings or even professional status were second consideration here this morning.

The nurse stepped away and defiantly crossed her arms across her chest in a physical act of complete disapproval.

"She could hurt herself if you let her pull her arm away," she said, in a last ditch effort to reassert some authority into the scene.

My sister in nursing didn't understand at all what was happening, right before her eyes. She should have been considered just too stupid to be allowed to practice nursing, especially pediatric nursing in the intensive care unit.

"If she says she won't move, she won't move," Patrick reminded her, again. This time a little more emphatically.

Patrick held Michele's arm gently, but solidly, so that the doctor could guide that big needle into that tiny, blue vein.

The needle pierced the skin Michele said, "Ouchie!" and closed her eyes tightly. She cried silently, squeezing a tear out of each eye as she closed them tightly to shut out the pain, but she didn't move. She squeezed my fingers with her other hand like a vise, but she didn't so much as flinch the arm with the needle.

In a few seconds the necessary blood was drawn, the needle removed and the wound pressed tightly with a sterile gauze pad that I reached over and handed to the doctor.

Dr. Kershnar told Michele how brave she was and what a good girl she had been. We already knew that, but it was nice to hear him tell her. He was very impressed with her courage.

"Tough kid."

I've often hoped that the nurse that day learned a lesson. She did, if she was paying any attention instead of just feeling sorry for herself — and feeling threatened — for having been pushed aside by Patrick. That one simple lesson could have made her a much better nurse for her patients. I'm afraid, however, that the lesson had been wasted on her. She was just too protective of her station. Too bad. I call it medical myopia.

If I could have a moment with every doctor — in fact with everyone who's involved with the delivery of health care services, I'd tell them to listen to your patients, even the very small ones. They almost always know more about themselves than you do. Don't even bother to ask how they are, unless you're willing to really listen to the answer they give you.

The young resident who asked Michele how she was, that first morning after surgery will never, ever asked a patient how they are again without listening closely to their response.

Remember, all of you in medicine, it's only partly science. The rest is part philosophy, part luck, some training, a little technique and a lot of intuition. It's also, in large part, the practice of simply paying attention.

At this point the three of us would like to make the following important point:

Always tell the truth — always. Never, ever lie to even the youngest patient. Remember, all of your patients are completely out of their natural element — suspended in a strange, alien world. They're on a spaceship, surrounded by unfamiliar sights and sounds. Their lives are in the hands of total strangers. If they are to trust these strangers, strangers who speak what seems to be another language, they must have the truth. The truth is the only lifeboat they have in this daunting world of fear and anxiety.

Who among us does not do better when we have the full knowledge of what's expected of us?

When we tell someone more than they can handle, they simply will not absorb the information. It's impossible to give a patient, no matter how young or how old, too much information.

Patsy has always been a good nurse, but after she was a patient, the daughter of a patient and then the mother of a patient, she became a much better nurse. As the song says, walk a mile in my shoes, if you want to know what it's like to be me.

Two days after the surgery we were walking out to the parking lot where we spotted Morton Woolley talking to another doctor. We cautiously approached. We still needed some answers to our questions, but we were still acting like this guy was seated next to God. I know it's irrational, but I also know it exists. I caution you to resist those feelings of inferiority if you possibly can, when you're in a situation like we were in during those dark days.

As we walked toward Woolley, he once again looked at us with a blank expression. He didn't have a clue who we were. Once again, we had to introduce ourselves.

Woolley offered us almost no information, answering our questions with abrupt, patronizing answers.

Did he have to remove a rib to get to the tumor? No. Did he think he'd gotten all of the cancer out? No. Some, because of the vital parts affected, had to be left in. What about those cells? It was hoped that radiation would destroy those cells.

Then, in a very condescending manner he said to the other doctor, as though Patsy wasn't standing right there, "Mrs. Nolan is one of our nurse mothers. She knows a little too much."

At that moment, I knew I hated this pathetic man. He might be considered by some to be the best pediatric surgeon in L.A., but he was one of the biggest horses asses I had ever met, anywhere. I am still embarrassed that I didn't confront him properly at that moment.

I excuse my timidity was basis on my anxiety for Michele's treatment at his hands. While I was willing to take on the nurse with the vice-like grip, the big cheese still had me intimidated, I'm sad to say. That's not an easy thing for me to admit. I have since been able to overcome that inherent veil of intimidation from the medical world, but on this day, in the parking lot at Childrens Hospital in Los Angeles, I actually thanked him for his time. Then I heard myself apologizing for interrupting him.

I've never really been able to excuse myself for the total lack of courage I displayed that day.

As we walked toward our car, I said to Patsy, under my breath so this paragon of surgical virtue couldn't possibly hear me, "That guy's the biggest jerk I've ever met."

"Yes, he sure is, but he's a hell of a surgeon."

For Michele, I knew which one was more important, but it didn't alter the fact that this guy was still as insensitive an egotistical jerk as had ever walked the planet.

For the next couple of days, Michele remained in ICU, battling for her life.

We discovered that the tumor had been attached to her adrenal gland and had completely encapsulated her right kidney, but we also found that there had been evidence of the malignancy in the renal artery. The tumor, the kidney, the adrenal gland had all been removed, along, at no extra charge, with her otherwise healthy appendix. The renal artery, however, would have to be treated with radiation.

The invasive, rapidly growing tumor had become so large that it had pushed its way up under her ribs. By the time they operated, the tumor was pressing up on her right lung, which had to be collapsed during surgery. A chest tube, connected to an external suction pump, had been inserted to help remove the air from her chest cavity as the collapsed lung expanded.

Twice a day, a respiratory therapist would come by and gently pound on her back to assist the collapsed lung in its effort to totally reinflate. My goodness it must be tough to know just how hard to pound, yet also know how much is too hard. Respiratory Therapists are seldom given enough credit for their talents and wonderful skills.

The first tube to be removed was her nose tube — she hated that one the worst. Then they took the foley out of her bladder, then the chest tube came out. The drain in her incision was still helping Michele's body heal from the inside out, so that tube stayed for a few more days. She was also down to just one IV in just one arm. Our baby was getting better.

The third day after Michele's operation, Patsy kept an appointment she'd made with her own doctor a week before Michele got sick.

"Are you okay?" I anxiously asked when she showed up at Childrens after the appointment.

"I'm fine. It's just that we're going to be parents again," she said, casually.

"You're kidding!"

"No, I was sure we were. I went to the doctor just to officially confirm what I already knew," she said.

God, I said, silently to myself, I sure hope we're not trading one kid for another here. It was a terrible thought to have cross one's mind, but cross my mind it did.

A few days later, as we walked from the parking lot to the front entrance of the hospital to see Michele, Patsy confided to me that she had experienced the same terrible thought about the new baby.

In truth, if you do lose a child and later have another baby, that new child doesn't replace one you lost. They are two disconnected acts. They are two completely different children.

So, if you lose a child, don't think you can replace the one who dies with a new baby. Have another baby if you like, but remember to let that new baby become a new person, not be a stand-in for the one you lost.

After her stay in ICU, Michele was moved to the nursery section of the hospital. She'd been in intensive care for four days. Her weight was down to just twenty-three pounds. Between the traumatic effects of the surgery, the debilitating effects of the cancer and the harsh invasion of the x-ray therapy, our happy, healthy, almost chubby little three year old was a pale skeleton of her former self. Skin and bones and deep sunken eyes were all you saw when you walked into her room.

That first night, as she rested comfortably in her own bed on the ward, we kissed her good night at eight o'clock, the end of regular visiting hours, and headed home. We explained that in ICU there were no visiting hours, they were always open for business, but here, where the children were not as sick as they were in ICU, we had to leave at eight so that the children could get their rest. We'd be back, we promised, first thing in the morning.

As with everything else that's explained so it can be clearly understood, she easily accepted this as a fact of life that couldn't be changed and never once asked us to stay or fussed when we left at the end of visiting hours.

On the other hand, we saw loving parents do unintentionally cruel things to their sick children. One lady, whose son was in the same ward with Michele, actually told me that it was just easier on them both when I asked her why she nightly told her son that she was going to the bathroom when she was actually leaving the hospital to go home.

"If I tell him I'm leaving, he cries and begs me to stay a little longer. If I just say I'm going to the bathroom he doesn't get upset. I hate to see him upset," she said.

"Let me tell you what happens after you leave. Your son waits and waits for you to come back, watching the door like a hawk. Finally, after about thirty minutes he starts asking the nurses what happened to his mommy. One of the nurses has to explain that mommy has gone home for the evening. Oh, no, she hasn't, he insists, she's just gone to the bathroom. It takes them an hour or more to calm him down and get him to go to sleep," I told her.

"How would you know? You always just say good night and leave. You're always gone before I am," she said as she tried to reject my comments.

"I know because the nurses have told me what happens, hoping I'll say something to you. It's not easier on your son and it's not easier on the nursing staff. Your son is probably having nightmares about his mommy falling into the toilet," I told her as gently as I could, putting my hand on her arm.

"What do you suggest? I hate to see him get upset when I have to leave," she said, pleading with me to help solve this dilemma for her.

"You can do what Patrick and I do for Michele. Explain the facts to him. Tell him the truth. Tell him that you love him. Tell him that you'll be back to feed him breakfast, but tell him that the rules say you have to leave at eight o'clock so that all the children can get their rest. The more rest he gets, the sooner he can go home, too. Then, kiss him good night without acting like you wish you could stay.

"Make leaving a normal, natural thing to do. He gets upset and anxious because he sees that you're upset and anxious about leaving. He's just following your lead. If you act like it's the right thing to do — if you accept it as being the proper thing to do — so will he," I advised her.

"But he's going to be upset and cry," she insisted.

"He may for the first night or two, but he won't be nearly as upset dealing with the truth as he has been dealing with your fibs," I told her.

"I do not lie to my son," she said with a little defensive anger in her voice.

"When you tell him you'll be right back, that you're only going down the hall to the bathroom, and then you go home and don't return until morning, you're lying to him. Not telling the truth is lying, and a lie is always more upsetting and much harder to deal with than the truth. Please, tell him the truth," I suggested.

"I just hate for him to cry," she said. "It's bad enough that he has to be in here."

"I know. It's not easy for any of us, but we're the grownups. We have to help them understand. If he understands why you have to leave, he'll probably accept it with out any fuss. At the very least, he won't think something terrible has happened to you in the bathroom. He's a very brave and a very smart little guy. He sees us leave Michele every night without any trouble. He'll quickly see that it's the thing for you to do, too."

That night we lingered a few minutes outside the ward to see how she did. I knew it was going to be hard for her to tell him she was going home.

She patiently told him it was time for her to go home for the night. She told him she loved him, she told him the nurses would take good care of him and then she said, "Good night," and kissed him.

Surprisingly, he reached his arms up, kissed her, hugged her and said, "Good night, mommy. I love you."

Patsy and the boy's mother walked to the elevator that night, together, with their arms around each other. Both were in tears. Being the mother of a child who's in the hospital, seriously ill, is not an easy job, even with another friendly and caring mother for support.

While it does help to have someone there who understands the pain and the heartache, it's still one of the hardest things a mother is ever asked to endure. If you're asked to be there for the mother of a sick child, remember, even as the child's father you cannot fully understand the primal connection that forever exists between a woman and her child. After all, they were connected, actually a part of each other, for those first nine months. It's real tough on mom when Susie's sick.

Even while Michele was still in the hospital, off she trucked, once a day, to radiation therapy as they aggressively attacked the cancer cells which remained like a time bomb within her tiny body. To help them direct the deadly beams of radiation precisely at the spots where they knew cancer cells were still lurking, they used a magic marker and drew lines right on the skin of her chest and stomach. She called the lines her "road map."

Those lines looked more like gun sights to me, but she didn't seem to mind them. She did, however, hate the radiation treatments. They not only made her sick to her stomach, but they completely destroyed her appetite. Even peanut butter, Cheerios and spaghetti were out. I never thought I'd see the day when she would turn down a plate of spaghetti.

We made a trip down to the office of the Chief of Radiology, Dr. Robert E. Hittle, to ask him a few questions. He was in charge of the therapy and seemed to be the one who would answer our questions. He gave us so much information, and in such a gentle manner. There should be more people like Dr. Hittle for parents to talk to about their child.

Dr. Hittle explained to me, when I asked about how much damage the radiation might be doing, that the x-rays in fact do strike a lot of healthy cells. It seems that one of the reasons they try so hard to be so precise about the direction of the beams is because they want to strike as few good cells as possible.

"You see," he told me, "The healthy cells and the cancer cells are both injured by the radiation. The healthy cells, because they are normal and healthy, recover from the ion bombardment. The cancer cells, on the other hand, are not as able to recover from the rays. That's why the trick in all of this is to give as much as is needed to blast those cancer cells out of there, yet stop short of doing too much damage to the healthy cells which happen to be in the line of fire."

Of course, her skin, which couldn't be missed by the rays, took on the appearance of paper thin, burnt leather. It became yellowish in places, brown in others. She would look, in just a few weeks, like she had been tanned the way leather is tanned. In effect, she had been.

Inside her tiny body, the microwaves were cooking parts of her as they smashed the cancer cells which were trying to kill her. It still seems a strange trade off, somehow.

The most important thing Dr. Hittle told us was, "You must hold Michele responsible for her actions just as you do her older sister. If you allow her to, she will use her illness to control you and she will become a tyrant. It's okay to tell a child no. Even a seriously ill child."

"Everything in medicine is a compromise of some kind," George Nardi, M.D., a wonderful physician and skilled surgeon would tell Patrick years later when I had to undergo gallbladder surgery.

"When you take a sharp scalpel and cut into a living human being, you're doing damage to that person. Repairable damage, but none the less, damage. Sometimes you're even doing serious damage. However, usually the damage inflicted by the surgeon is more than offset by the overriding need to remove or correct something that's killing the patient or causing serious pain or discomfort. But, it's still a compromise.

"We're going to do some damage to Patsy this morning, no question about it. But it's the only way we can get that diseased gallbladder out of her."

Today, of course, there are new developments in surgery and many times extensive, invasive surgery can be avoided, like the new techniques in treatment of a diseased gallbladder.

Since George Nardi told me that, I've had a better time dealing with all the damage we did to Michele over those first two horrible years. It helped, but it still didn't make remembering that charred, paper thin skin on the body of our three year old a whole lot easier.

Since I feel strongly that we should point out the people who gave Michele and her parents less than their best, I feel we should also remind you of those who gave great care — sometimes even exceptional care and understanding to Michele and to her parents.

There are a lot of people we wish to thank for their outstanding service to our daughter, but there's one guy I want you to know.

I had been so impressed with the gentle care the big nurses aid in ICU had given to Michele — and to all the other kids he cared for, that I wanted to do something nice for him. Something special. I guessed that he might just be a football fan.

I enjoyed a certain amount of pull with the sales department at the television station, so a few days before the Los Angeles Rams — Chicago Bears NFL football game at the Los Angeles Memorial Coliseum I called in an I.O.U. I wrangled two tickets in the tenth row, on the press box side, right smack dab on the fifty yard line out of Sales. These are among the best seats in the Coliseum.

That afternoon, on my way to see Michele, I went up to ICU and there he was, helping a small child.

"Are you a Ram fan by any chance?," I asked him.

"Sure am, but I don't get a chance to see them very much."

He smiled at me with that warm smile of his, as he was carefully replacing a spoiled bandage on a tiny tot of about four.

I teased him a little more, and he knew I was teasing, "You probably have to work this Sunday?"

"I work most of the time. I've got six kids."

"Well, that's too bad," I said as I pulled out the two precious tickets to the sold out football game.

"I just happen to have two extra tickets on the fifty yard line to this week's Bears game and I can't find anyone who can use them. If you're scheduled to work Sunday, you won't be needing them either, will you?" I teased.

"I think I can make arrangements to get off the schedule this Sunday," he said with a big grin.

I winked at him, hugged his massive shoulders and tucked the tickets into the pocket of his scrub suit.

"Have a great time. I hope the Rams win, but if they don't, have a good time anyway," I said.

He was very pleased to get the tickets. "Thank you very much."

"No! Thank you. Thank you for taking such great care of all these little people. I'll never be able to say enough about the way you gave our Michele such special treatment."

He looked down at the tiny patient in the bed before him and quietly said, "Just doing my job."

"No, you're doing more than just your job. You're saving lives and more than that, you're giving exceptional care to a lot of very sick, very scared kids and their parents. You should get a medal and a big raise, not two dumb tickets to a football game," I told him.

"Maybe one day you'll write a book about your daughter and you can mention me in it," he said, continuing to gently apply the new dressing to the child.

He chuckled softly and thanked me again for the tickets.

Before I slipped out of ICU, his face grew serious as he asked, "How's Michele doing?"

"Thanks to you and the rest of the nurses and aides at this hospital, she's getting better every day. I think we're going to take her home on Wednesday."

"That's great. Say, are you sure you don't want to go to the game on Sunday?"

"Are you kidding? I've got to be here Sunday. I have to cover for you."

He smiled.

"Have a swell time," I said.

As I left ICU, he waved one huge hand and flashed another of those big, gold-filled smiles. This was one terrific man. May all of us get the care he gives when we're in need.

I've done my best to remember his name, without success. The personnel records at Childrens hospital could only give me a couple of possible names, since there were several people with the same description working that day, and I don't want to give credit here to the wrong person. I know who he was, and what he meant to us twenty-five years ago, and I just hope he recognizes himself in these pages.

I still feel good just thinking about that guy.

... as the founder and director of the Jimmy Fund in Boston,
Dr. Sidney Farber had been an early leader in the successful treatment of
Wilm's tumor. The Jimmy Fund kids enjoyed the best survival record
in the country — which meant in the world.
Boston would be just fine for Michele, I concluded.
I wasn't as sure about me and the baby, however.

Chapter Five

A Guy In Boston Called Today!

I spent the days after the operation trying to juggle the work at KHJ-TV, see that Patsy and Michele got whatever they needed at the hospital, while finding time to assure Teresa that we hadn't abandoned our oldest child.

I went to the hospital for a few minutes each morning on my way to the studio, returning after work to spend the evening with Michele. Patsy was there from morning until the end of visiting hours. Thank goodness we had the help of Patsy's wonderful and loving mom, during those stressful days.

Lillian Whalen was terrific during those awful days, making dinner each night and raising all of our spirits. It always made people feel better just to be around Patsy's sweet mom.

Lillian, the mother of Patsy and the grandmother of Michele was experiencing a double pain. All the while suffering silently. While she was terribly concerned about the health of her granddaughter, she was almost equally concerned about the pain her own daughter was experiencing during this ordeal. It was a while before I began to understand her special anguish.

Today, as I recall my behavior during that time, I don't think I was very sensitive to mom's pain. Although, in later years, when I attempted to apologize to her for my lack of sensitivity during the time Michele was sick, mom, of course, denied that I had been thoughtless in her regard. She may have dismissed it, after the fact, but I know I wasn't as attuned to her needs and apprehensions as I should have been — or could have been. Even though she's gone now, I still want to say to her, Sorry, mom. I could have done better.

I may have been too wrapped up in what I was personally experiencing and worrying about when I should have been more tuned in to the fears and the mental and emotional anguish which this gentle, loving woman was being asked to quietly accept. I made the mistake of expecting her to just be there, a strong, willing and understanding grandmother. She was all that and more, but she undoubtedly needed more loving care than I gave her during those frightening days. We talked about the disease, of course, and she visited Michele in the hospital, but I should have spent more time comforting Patsy's mom than I did.

Twenty years later, when Lillian quietly slipped from our lives, a few short hours after experiencing a massive stroke, I was asked by her children to deliver her eulogy. It remains to this day my greatest honor. As I sat down to write what I would say at her funeral mass, I knew that I would never be able to put into words how much this wonderful woman had meant to me, or how much she had meant to her entire family.

I knew that she had touched everyone who had ever known her. I knew, in my heart, that I would never, ever be able to put into any of the words in the English language what this dear, sweet, wonderful, loving lady had meant to my life for over three decades. I did know that she had loved me deeply for over thirty years. To her, whatever I said or did was just fine.

With that strength in my heart — a strength which she had helped place there — I let my heart write what I would say to them as her family gathered together to pay their final respects at her service in Reno.

I ended my remarks the day we laid her to rest by saying through my tears, what I will say it as long as I draw breath, "She was the best any of us would ever know."

Not only had Patsy's mom accepted me, unconditionally, as the choice her daughter had made in a husband, but she took me into her heart with all the love she would have had for a child she had borne.

I shall always miss her soft touch, warm voice and kind words. I miss her non judgmental council, her delicious sense of humor and her love. I cannot explain the wonderful feeling of peace which I know existed between us. I never concluded a telephone conversation or walked away from her after a personal visit without telling her that I loved her. She never failed to tell me she loved me, too. I miss her terribly, even to this day. I will miss her until the day I die.

Taking over in our critical hour of need during Michele's first surgery, without complaint, without hesitation, was just one of the loving things that this near perfect woman did for me in the third of a century of mutual love and devotion we experienced together. Lillian Whalen was not only the best mother-in-law anyone will ever have, she was indeed the best person any of us will ever know.

None of us can appreciate the depths of the pain nor the extent of the heartache Patsy's mom experienced during Michele's illness. I know, having known her so well, that her pain was intense, but she held it within herself — as did my own mom, to a certain extent.

Being an extremely private person, Patsy's mom only expressed those personal thoughts, fears and feelings with her God.

I do know that the fear of losing Michele was a very great fear with her. In later years, she and I would talk about the loss of a child. She was the last of thirteen children, eleven of whom lived into their eighties — she survived all but one. Just think: eleven times she had to bear the news that one of her brothers or one of her sisters had died.

One time, ten years after Michele's first surgery, I was on a trip from our home in Boston to the west coast. On the way home, I made a slight detour so I could stop in Boulder City, Nevada and have dinner with my mother-in-law. It was only a few months after Patsy's dad, Luke, had died.

Rather than go out somewhere to dinner, mom and I decided to spend the evening at home, just the two of us. We talked about the kids, about the many joys our mates had brought us. I was a wonderful evening in which we laughed at a number of silly things.

Sometime during the evening, we began to talk about the things we found difficult to share with others, even with our own family. It was then, as we sat at the table during this, one of our most personal talks, that she told me of a well remembered, grief-filled experience when she was an eleven-year-old child.

It seems that Tommy Hastings, one of her older brothers, had been born with crippled legs (spina bifida, she thought perhaps, but she didn't really know because things like that were not openly discussed with children in those days).

Tommy never was able to walk. He had to use crutches to get around. His baby sister, Lillian, many times acted as his hands — and in some cases, his legs. She would carry things for him, run errands around the farm for him and do a lot of things that her healthy, strong legs could easily do when his useless legs could not.

While her brother Joe remained throughout her life her very favorite sibling, Lillian had a special fondness for her crippled brother, Tommy.

When Lillian was eleven, quite suddenly, Tommy died. It happened just after he had celebrated his twenty-first birthday.

Tommy's death was a great shock to Lillian.

That night, as we sat there in the kitchen in Boulder City, more than fifty years after his death, Lillian told me that everyone in her family was so busy with their own feelings of grief and guilt that they didn't have much time to deal with the grief of a skinny little girl of eleven. She said she was forced to face her grief without much help from the others in her family. It was a very hard experience for a young girl.

Lillian told me that it was that experience, the experience of not being able to successfully deal with her grief which influenced her decision to always hold on to her feelings — particularly her feelings of sadness or loss. Since the days of Tommy's death, Lillian had always kept the tears deep within her self, never letting the pain out. She never allowed herself to express sad emotions in public or even in front of other members of the family.

During the more than thirty years that I knew and loved her, I only saw my mother-in-law cry on two occasions. One of them was that night as we sat at her kitchen table in Boulder City, talking about Tommy. Talk about someone with a stiff upper lip!

On the other hand, Lillian's feelings of joy and happiness were shared with all of us — she was generally a very happy and cheerful person. She could make us all laugh.

But she did not often share, even with her husband Luke, her feelings of sadness, fear or despair. To her, the outward expression of grief was merely an attempt to call attention to your own pain. And Lillian believed that one's pain was to be dealt with privately, internally.

One time, early in our marriage, Patsy was visiting her folks. I had not been able to accompany her, but, instead, I had joined her the next day. I had the unfortunate duty to bring my bride the sad news of the suicide of one of my early mentors in the broadcast business. He was a man who I had greatly admired and respected. Art Sprinkle's death was completely senseless.

As Patsy and I stood in Lillian's kitchen, softly crying together over the frustrating loss of our friend, my mother-in-law gently scolded us both for letting our emotions spill over into the preparations for dinner, there in the middle of the kitchen. Lillian thought we should have chosen a more private place to console each other. And she was probably correct. But Patsy and I have never been ashamed of our expressions of sadness or affection. As I have said, Lillian was only a near-perfect person.

Years after that, as Lillian and I sat at the kitchen table in Boulder City, she also told me of how much she missed her partner in life, Patsy's dad, Luke. She talked lovingly of the man with whom she had shared her life for over forty years. Suddenly her eyes filled with tears as she reached out to take my hand.

Squeezing my hand tightly, she said, "Oh, Patrick, sometimes I feel like I can just reach right out and touch him."

The tears were there because she loved him so much and could no longer just reach right out and touch him. For her to share those deep feelings with me did, of course, make an everlasting impression on me.

The only other time I saw her cry was on that emotion filled evening when she arrived at our house the night before Michele's first surgery. Mom walked into our living room, directly from the airport, desperate to somehow ease the pain and reduce the fears she knew had to be nearly overwhelming her oldest daughter. I have never seen a more painful look on anyone's face — before or since. The feelings which were reflected on that good woman's face were intense.

"Oh, Patsy Ann, my dear," she said, as she took her daughter in her arms, "What can I do?"

I loved my "other" mom very much and there is hardly a day that I don't think of her with great fondness. Both Patsy and I miss her a great deal.

Thank you for loving me, Lillian Whalen. I will always love you and treasure your gift of love — a gift that you began to give me on the first day we met.

It should be noted here, that as the years have passed, Michele has been known to sometimes conceal her emotions, in much the same way as her Grandma Whalen often did. As a friend to both, I'm happy to report that in a variety of wonderful ways a lot of her maternal Grandma can be found in Michele's character.

Both Lillian Whalen and Michele Nolan were born with pure hearts. They will always be two of my greatest treasures.

During the time Michele was in the hospital, Patrick, doing most of the work on just one weekend, built her a pink playhouse. It had windows, a door, even a second story sun deck. He found some huge plastic, yellow sunflower decals and put them all over the playhouse. It was quite a happy, colorful homecoming present for her.

The day we brought Michele home from the hospital, she insisted on walking out to the back yard, right from the car, to see her "house". She said it hurt too much to have Patrick carry her, so she walked. She walked all bent over, a little like Groucho Marx, only very slowly. She walked down the driveway in her soft, pink bathrobe and into the back yard to see her new playhouse. She loved the house. It was a good tonic for her. Those huge blue eyes finally showed a little brightness for the first time in two weeks.

The first evening home from the hospital, Michele was standing in front of the sofa. She looked up at me, her big eyes so sad as she said, "Mama, look, I can't even hop!"

After a delicate hug and my reassurance that her "hop" would return before long, she felt a little better, but she still wished she could hop.

The days that followed saw daily trips to the hospital for radiation treatments. Five days a week, for six weeks, we would drive to the hospital, Michele would bravely walk into the Radiation Therapy department, lay flat on a table for 30 to 60 minutes and be given her radiation therapy.

Five days a week, the first week of each month, we would go to the clinic for her chemotherapy. During those visits, I became aware of the human mind's capacity for survival. There is always someone who is worse off than you. With that in mind, I knew I could survive anything.

I remember a woman from England, a lovely woman in her early forties, who had three-year-old twin daughters. These two beautiful children were her only children, and would be her only children. She told me that she was unable to bear any more children.

It nearly broke my heart when she told me that both of these lovely girls had leukemia. Our problem seemed to be so simple. After all, they could cut the tumor out of Michele. You can't remove leukemia with a scalpel.

The last time I talked to that woman she was making final plans to return to England. She told me that she had family there for support and socialized medicine for the girls. The woman couldn't afford, emotionally or financially, to remain in Los Angeles any longer. I've often wondered how things worked out for her and for the twins. I hope they're able to read Michele's story. I hope they are all well.

Since I had not been a permanent employee for the required length of time, we did not yet have coverage under the company health insurance. I knew we were looking at a big bill from both the hospital as well as the doctors. We knew they were both going to be monsters.

On one of the first days after Michele was admitted to the hospital, Milt Hoffman called me into his office. Hugh Delregno, the company's comptroller at KHJ-TV, and Milt had had a little meeting.

It seems that when I joined the station as the summer weekend director, I was listed on the payroll as a temporary employee — per diem, no benefits. A few months later, when they gave me the job as Producer of Tempo, I was promoted to full-time, regular employee status. The coverage, however, would not cover Michele's illness because the family hadn't been covered for the required ninety days when she went to the hospital.

Milt said that he and Hugh had decided to make a few retroactive mathematical corrections, for insurance purposes. They had decided to move my full time employment date back four months. After all, as Milt said, I had been working like a full time employee, all along, I might as well get some of the benefits.

"Besides," Milt said, "we don't want to have to take up an office collection to bail you out of jail."

I've always been deeply indebted to both Milt and Hugh for their thoughtfulness. They had each taken a big, personal risk for us. They had risked being in a lot of trouble with both management and the insurance company, but they hadn't let that stop them from doing what they could to help us. It was a wonderful, courageous thing for both of them to have done. I'll never forget either one of those guys. I have no fear of telling that story now. The statute of limitations has long ago run out!

Although I have no evidence, I've always strongly felt that my pal, Walt Baker, who was the production manager at the time and who would later serve as Vice-President of Programming for the station, had had a hand in this little "date correction" business, too. I have no proof and Walt's always denied having any involvement, but I'm still not convinced he wasn't in on it.

The insurance paid for a great deal of the hospital charges, but not Woolley's bill. More on how I handled that in a later chapter.

As the next few weeks passed, the first course of radiation treatments ended, Patsy's mom went back home to Boulder City and things at the Nolan house got back to some semblance of normal, but they didn't stay that way for long.

One day at work, a day where everything that could go wrong had gone wrong, I was talking on the phone to a publicist who worked out of her home on Cape Cod. Abby was telling me how beautiful it could be there in New England and I was feeling stressed out over a particularly difficult week of poor shows in Los Angeles.

"Why don't you find me a job back there, Abby. I'll move back to Massachusetts and we can watch the sunrise together one day in Hyannis," I said, almost casually.

As it turned out, that became one of the most important conversation I ever had with anyone. Without that casual conversation on the phone, with a person I only knew on the phone and would never, as it turned out, ever meet in person, Michele probably would not have survived.

I talked to Abby toward the end of the day on a Thursday. The next morning, soon after arriving at the office, I took a call from Squire Derrick Rushnell, executive producer at WBZ-TV, in Boston. Even though he had a title for a first name, Squire sounded like a real nice guy on the phone. He was warm, friendly and relaxed.

He asked me a few questions and then he said, without bothering to find out if I was even interested, "We'd like you to fly to Boston this weekend and talk to us about producing our new morning talk show. There's a ticket waiting for you at the American Airlines counter at LAX. You're booked on tonight's red eye to Logan. In the morning, when you get in, take a cab to the Sheraton Copley, there's a room reserved for you, in your name. I'll call you at the Copley about nine tomorrow morning."

"Squire," I said,"Can I call you back in a few minutes? I'd like to touch bases with Patsy before I run clear across the country for the weekend."

"Sure. I'll be here for another half hour or so. Here's my direct number," he said as he gave me the number of his private line.

"I'll see you in the morning. Have a nice flight. Oh, by the way, does the red eye give you any trouble?"

"Squire, I've never been east of Chicago. I don't know if the red eye's a problem for me or not. I've never been on it."

Squire rang off and I called Patsy. She said it was a good opportunity to see Boston in the winter.

That night I caught the plane to Boston. The flight didn't bother me. In fact, I rather enjoyed the first of what would become a great many red eye special flights across the country for me.

While Patrick was in Boston, I talked to the people at Childrens Hospital. I didn't want to disrupted Michele's treatments by flying off to the other side of the country, just to follow a good career move for Patrick. And, of course, neither did Patrick.

The radiation therapist, Dr. Hittle, told me that they would prefer we not take Michele anywhere for two years, but that if we did move, the only place we could go that was just as good a place as Los Angeles for Michele would be Boston.

Closely associated with Childrens Hospital in Boston is a clinic known as The Jimmy Fund. The Jimmy Fund has been a world leader in the treatment of children's cancer, leukemia and Wilm's tumor being the two most common.

When Jackie Jensen — who would later become a good friend of Patsy;'s brother Brian Whalen at the University of Nevada — and Ted Williams had been stars with the Boston Red Sox in the forties, the Jimmy Fund became the major charitable organization of the ball club. Williams raised millions of dollars for the Jimmy Fund, always without a single shred of personal publicity.

Today the Jimmy Fund is officially been renamed The Dana Farber Cancer Foundation. It continues to do its important, lifesaving work with children. A portion of the profits from the sale of this story are earmarked for the Jimmy Fund. It won't be as much as Ted Williams raised and contributed over the years, but it's what our family can do to say, Thanks.

The late founder and first director of the Jimmy Fund in Boston, Dr. Sidney Farber, had been an early leader in the successful treatment of Wilm's tumor. The Jimmy Fund kids enjoyed the best survival record in the country — which meant in the world. Boston would be just fine for Michele, I concluded.

I wasn't as sure about me and the new baby, however.

In Los Angeles, we had just located a wonderful young OBGYN who just loved helping people have babies. He had developed one of the first "Birthing Centers" in the nation. It was like a motel, with private rooms for the family during labor. The rooms were warm, comfortable places with table lamps and carpet and real furniture instead of fluorescent ceiling lights, linoleum and hard chairs. Not only was it a wonderful place to have a baby, but, if you and the baby were doing fine, you went home the same day. I was really looking forward to having this new baby without a huge fight between Patrick and the medical world.

Dr. Ed had eagerly included Patrick in the process, right from the very first office visit. Patrick was really looking forward to this pregnancy and ultimately to the birth of his third child.

Now here we were, faced with the possibility of another major move while I was pregnant. I wanted to stay in L.A., get Michele well and have this new baby, without the hassles of moving again, particularly clear across the country. But, alas, I knew in my heart that it was not to be.

Boston overwhelmed me. I had never been to a city like this before. I was almost instantly in love.

I took the call from Squire about an hour after I got to the hotel. In another hour I found myself in the office of the Vice-President of Westinghouse Broadcasting, Win Baker, talking about a new morning talk show they were planning to develop. It was a major career opportunity. I was dying to take a crack at it.

"Did you talk to the doctors?" I asked Patsy when I called after the meeting.

"Yes. They said that if we want to move to Boston it will not put Michele in any jeopardy. In fact, Boston is the best place for her type of cancer to be treated. So, if they offer you the job, don't let our concerns for Michele influence you. Michele will be just fine in Boston. I'm not sure I will be, but Michele will be fine."

"What do you mean, you're not sure about you?"

"I just dread the thought of another major move. Patrick, remember, I'm just a little pregnant," she said.

"I've already talked to them about that. If they offer me the job, and if I take it, they will move us, period. You won't pack or unpack a single box. They'll send the guys with the big truck and you and the girls will walk out the door with only a suitcase in your hands."

"Promise?"

"Absolutely. I'm telling you. That part of the deal is non negotiable or there's no deal," I quickly assured her.

An hour later, Mel Bernstein, the program director — and Squire's boss — called to offer me the job. I negotiated a salary figure and then reminded him of our moving discussions.

"Mel, my wife is five months pregnant and she moves nothing. Either our deal includes the total expenses of moving our family or we have no deal."

Mel assured me that the company would pay for the entire move. He told me to just hurry up and get back here in two weeks, we had lots of work to do.

I called Patsy back and told her to pack her suitcase, we were moving to New England. I rang off and went for a four hour walking tour of my new city.

I knew we were going to love it in Boston and I knew we were going to be very happy there, too.

In truth, I wasn't thinking too much about Michele or her illness. This was by now the middle of February and it had been over six months since the surgery. The fear of losing her was substantially reduced and I was looking forward to this new adventure in New England with great anticipation. I was booked home on an early Sunday morning flight. I couldn't wait to get home to tell Patsy and Teresa and Michele about Boston.

After a great meal at the hotel — on Westinghouse, of course — I went to bed Saturday night still suffering a little jet lag, but smiling from ear to ear. A new, exciting job, a new exciting city and soon, a new baby. I'm sure it was well after midnight before I finally drifted off to sleep.

In the morning, I took my wake up call, sprang out of bed and took a peak out the window. I was on the sixth floor, but I couldn't see the ground. I couldn't see the sky, either. In fact, all I could see was white. It was snowing like crazy and had apparently been doing so for hours. There was a lot of snow out there. I'd never been sixty feet up in a snow storm before.

I hurriedly called my airline. Sorry, they said, all flights in and out of Boston have been canceled — indefinitely . Didn't I know there was a major winter snow storm in Boston, they asked. Yep! I knew. Now I knew.

What about New York, I asked. Was the storm affecting flights out of New York?

No, I was told. New York is clear and operating as usual. Great, I said, book me on an afternoon flight for L.A. out of JFK. I'll take the train to New York.

I called the train station. I could get a train to New York in about an hour. They said the Back Bay Station was just across Copley Square from my hotel. I would be in New York by one thirty. My flight was at four. I was excited. Not only was I going home, I would get my first look at New York City and I'd have a wonderful four hour train ride down the coast and through the New England countryside ... snow and all. I love train trips. What a weekend this was turning out to be, I thought, cheerfully. Little did I know what kind of an adventure lay ahead of me.

The train pulled out a few minutes late, but I wasn't worried. There was still plenty of time to make my afternoon flight. During the hours that followed our departure from Boston, I learned all about New England's unpredictable weather.

By the time the train pulled into Providence, the storm showed no signed of abating. In fact, if anything, it was snowing harder in Rhode Island than it had been in Boston.

By the time we reached Hartford, the switches were frozen — most of them in a closed position. In Bridgeport, the bridge was frozen — open. We sat there, completely stopped, for over an hour. We were now running about two hours late. I knew by this time that I would have to get a later flight to L.A. Maybe, I thought, there was the possibility of catching a red eye in the other direction.

By the time we reached New Haven, the train was packed to the ceiling with people, all trying to get to New York. The planes weren't flying. Buses weren't running. Cars were being abandoned everywhere. That day, our train was the only thing, it seemed, moving toward the Big Apple. We moved very slowly through the storm as thne storm was moving south.

At every stop, another herd of impatient people clambered aboard the crowded train, with their suitcases, boxes and bags. Before long the isles in all the cars were jammed with people standing everywhere, sitting on their suitcases or waiting to steal someone's seat. You didn't dare get up to go to the rest room or to the snack bar because when you came back to your seat it would be occupied. Long before we arrived at Penn Station, I knew I would not be flying into the setting sun on this particular winter day.

As often happens in times of shared adventures, everyone seems drawn a little closer to the others involved. Strangers become instant friends. I made a friendship on that trip that endures to this day.

I spent almost that entire trip sitting with an airline pilot who was trying to get to Kennedy to fly his own flight out. The pilot and I were sitting directly across from, and facing, a young woman who worked for IBM and Betsy Hirsch (later to be Katz), a first year college student at Boston University. Although we haven't seen each other for several years, Betsy and I remain good friends to this day, corresponding several times a year. Happily married now, Betsy and her husband Al have two beautiful children. They live in Reading, Pennsylvania.

In Hartford, we were delayed while they switched from a diesel engine to an electric engine because as the train from New England approaches the city, it goes underground before it reaches the East River. The tracks at Penn Station are, after all, underground.

There in the dark tunnel, away from the storm, things didn't seem to be so bleak, but when we came up to the street from the underground tracks at Penn Station, we walked onto a world of pure white. Heavy snow was falling in huge flakes and the wind was blowing it around our faces and into our eyes. The storm had just followed the train down the east coast to New York City. It was quite a memorable introduction to Manhattan, I can tell you.

IBM and Betsy were both met on the platform when we arrived. Betsy's parents and IBM's husband had been waiting for hours for our train to arrive. We were over six hours late.

We said our goodbyes to IBM and Betsy and their folks and then the pilot and I walked off down a snowy New York street, without much of a plan. After walking a couple of blocks, we stumbled into the lobby of the New York Hilton.

I stayed at the Hilton as the storm raged outside over New York City. Three days later, with the help of a friend I met at the airport, I managed to catch the first flight out of JFK after the terrible storm. It had been quite an adventure, but there was still a lot more traveling fun in store for me this particular winter.

Two weeks later, we packed our suitcases, gave the keys to the house to the movers and caught a plane to Las Vegas. The girls and I would spend a couple of weeks with my folks in Boulder City while Patrick went on ahead to start his new job and find a house for our growing family. The girls and I would wait in Boulder City while the truck full of our things made the long, winter trip across the country. Patrick had even arranged to have one of the mover's drive his Mustang to Boston. Trading in the family station wagon in Los Angeles, we had arranged to pick up a new car at the factory in Michigan in a few weeks. Ready or not, Boston — here we come.

Patrick stayed with us in Boulder City through the weekend. On Sunday, I drove him to McCarran Field in Las Vegas.

84

On his trip to Boston, he was taking with him everything he would need for the two weeks before our moving van arrived, including a big tropical Angel fish. Patrick had made a wager with a friend that he could get the tropical fish to Boston, in the dead of winter, alive. Here he was, traveling clear across the country, loaded down with all his television stuff and a tropical fish in his carry on suitcase. It was not the craziest thing that he's done since we've been married, but it sure was close to the craziest. The wager, by the way, was five bucks!

While Patrick and his fish flew off into the snow and cold of the east, the girls and I would have two restful, warm and very pleasant weeks in Boulder City with my folks.

Although my dad had always said that visiting relatives and fish are both only good for about three days, the girls and I had a lovely visit. Teresa and Michele played in the park under the watchful eye of their mother who was growing ever larger each day with the new baby.

Michele, it seemed, was getting a little stronger each day. The radiation had taken a terrible toll on her system, but she's such a scrappy little kid that she never, ever gave in to it. She might not be able to keep up with the much more athletic and vigorous Teresa, but she would just keep running until she got there. Teresa could climb to the top of the jungle gym in a few seconds. Michele's climb took several minutes, but she never complained that Teresa was ahead of her. She seemed, somehow, to completely understand that if she did the best she could do, that it would be just fine. She's always done the very best she can do — at everything — even though it might take a bit longer.

Those days in Boulder City were quite restful, but a little lonely. Patrick was twenty-five hundred miles away and I missed him. He called every night to talk to us, but it wasn't the same as actually having him right there with us. I knew he missed the three of us, terribly, as well.

There Patrick was, alone in a strange town, with a new, stress filled job, far from his family. He wanted his girls to be there when he came home at night, but every night he came home to an empty hotel room at the Copley Plaza Hotel. Empty, that is, except for a large tropical fish who was living in a converted ice bucket under a disassembled hotel table lamp. Patrick won, but he never collected the five dollar bet.

Patrick hung a huge sign over the ice bucket for the housekeeping staff, in both English and Spanish, that said, Do Not Touch — Live Fish — Pelegro!

The story of that "fish adventure," all carried out in the dead of winter with diverted flights, unscheduled hotel stops, taxi cabs, motel rooms, ice buckets and a series of borrowed electrical plugs which were needed to periodically fill the fish's plastic bag with air and borrowed from behind airline ticket counters from hassled and surprised clerks, would fill a book of it's own. Remember, it was all done for a silly five dollar bet, which was never paid. (That fish did live for another two years after it arrived in Boston, however.)

While we were in Boulder City, the girls and I went down to visit Hoover Dam, with my dad who had helped build it. In many places the dam is still called Boulder Dam by a lot of Roosevelt Democrats.

We didn't take the usual three hour tour of the dam that my father loved to lead visiting friends and relatives through, because Michele just tired too easily and I wasn't able to carry her very far in my condition. Michele might weigh less than thirty pounds, but the child growing in my womb was getting bigger each day.

However, my condition didn't stop Teresa and her granddad. Leaving Michele and me behind at the top, they were able to explore some of the seldom visited caves and tunnels deep within one of the eight engineering wonders of the world. They both had a grand time. My father loved to show off, "his dam."

The only sad thing that happened to us during those two weeks was the loss of our family dog who had been given to Patrick when she was a small pup by a friend. JoJo was a Puli, a breed of sheep dog that's very intelligent and wonderful with children. She would let the kids fall on her, pull her long hair and never once growl or bark or even show any discomfort or unhappiness.

As often happens with most of these dogs, JoJo was heavily imprinted on one member of the family. We all recognized that JoJo was, by her own choosing, Patrick's dog. She could identify the sound of his car when it was a block away and jump up to be waiting at the door for him. I tested her, and, sure enough, she knew he was coming before I could see his car down the street. JoJo was an amazing animal.

One day, while we were at mom and dad's, she must have decided to go looking for Patrick. In the past, if he was away from home for more than two days she would get very nervous and would anxiously listen for the sound of his car.

This day, in Boulder City, she jumped over the back fence and went, I believe, in search of Patrick. Since Boulder City is a tourist town, I'm sure she was picked up by someone who was visiting for the day. She still had on her L.A. dog tag and the people who found her probably never thought to check with the local authorities about a missing dog. She was very friendly and would go to anyone. She probably just climbed into a stranger's car and was out of town before we even noticed she was out of the yard. I waited three days, hoping she would turn up or that our town wide searches would produce a shaggy brown dog named JoJo, but it didn't.

Finally, I had to call Boston and tell Patrick that JoJo was among the missing. It nearly killed me to tell him about JoJo. I don't think he's ever forgiven me for losing his dog on that trip.

A few days later, the girls and I were on the plane headed for our new adventure in New England.

While the big moving truck plowed through the snow and ice of winter, I was stuck trying to find a house for my family that would be ready to move into when our furniture pulled into town. Since we were working on the new show until eight or so every night — and still trying to deliver the existing show every morning — I was reduced to searching for a house on the one weekend I would have before the furniture arrived. I knew if I didn't find a place during that tiny window of opportunity I would have to try to get all that stuff into my room on the twelfth floor at the Sheraton with the fish. I didn't think the bell captain was going to like that job.

Jerry Williams, a guy who does talk shows for the highest bidder, was working for WBZ at that time. He told me that there was a charming little village about twenty miles out to the west of Boston where the schools were good, the people were mostly friendly and the commute was fairly easy. WBZ is located just off the Turnpike on the west side of Boston, just across the river from Harvard. It's actually almost next door to Harvard Stadium, which is, interestingly enough, not in Cambridge, or Middlesex County where the University is located, but across the mighty Charles River, in Boston, Suffolk County — from whence came the hated British on that fateful night back in 1775.

Jerry said that I should drive out to this historic little village that can trace its roots all the way back to 1637 — a hundred and thirty-eight years before the famous midnight ride of Paul Revere — and which has been, since that early year, a functioning democratic form of government, from that day to this. Sudbury, Massachusetts has been governed by a Town Meeting form of government for over three hundred years. One man (and eventually, one woman, too), one vote. Every registered voter in the town is a member of the town's legislative body — the Annual Town Meeting.

On Saturday morning, bright and early, I drove my borrowed station car, on loan from the news department, out of the Sheraton underground garage and onto the clear, dry Massachusetts Turnpike. The snow, crisp and white, was piled ten feet high on both the sides of the road as my inconspicuous orange and white station wagon sped along the turnpike while displaying huge black and white letters along each side proclaiming, for all to see, that here was an important member of the Eyewitness News Team. The forest of scanners and two way radio antennas on the roof, the Emergency Road Kit in the back window and the giant WBZ on the hood, tailgate and roof, allowed me to quietly slip, completely unnoticed, into Sudbury.

For me, Sudbury was love at first sight.

Sudbury is still a very special place for me. I spent the third decade of my life in that quite little village of American history and New England charm.

I turned in at the first real estate office I came to. I was met by a bright, good looking young man who said that, yes, there were some places available.

"Does it have to have trees?" was one of his first curious questions.

"It only has to have a good furnace and at least one indoor bathroom," I said. "My wife doesn't like the cold and she's almost six months pregnant."

We looked at several nice New England houses, all of them out of our price range. Finally, he turned off The Boston Post Road on to Horse Pond Road.

"I have a great idea," he said. "There's a fellow down here with a house that's tied up in a divorce. He's planning to sell, but he can't put it on the market until he makes a property settlement with his wife. It's a real messy divorce. I think I can get him to lease it to you with an option to buy it when the divorce is final. Neither one of them wants the house, and it would be perfect for your family."

We turned off of Horse Pond Road into a narrow, snow filled road called, Old Meadow Road. At the very end of the road sat a single story, white, four bedroom house. There was a path shoveled up to the front porch from the driveway through the six feet of snow which had accumulated on the front lawn.

In a very few minutes the landlord, who was there at the time, and I, had struck a deal. A two year lease with an option to buy when the divorce court ordered the house sold and the proceeds divided. I'd been in town for two hours and we had a place to live. I called Boulder City and told Patsy the good news — we had a house. She was greatly relieved.

"Now," she said, somewhat sarcastically, "all I have to do is unpack all those damn boxes when we get there."

I remained silent.

I spent the rest of the day driving around the narrow, snow banked roads of Sudbury, getting to know our new town. The more I saw of Sudbury, the more I loved this quaint New England village.

Now, where was that big truck with all our stuff?

All I needed now was that truck and my girls.

Later that night, back at the Sheraton, I ordered a big bottle of champagne, a thick, rare steak, which, of course, I charged to Westinghouse. Boston was going to be a great place to live I thought. I was getting into a very mellow mood. The only problem I still had was trying to figure out what I was going to do with my free Sunday.

Patsy has a built in device that lets her "know" certain things. It was probably turned on the night Michele went to the doctor and Pasty knew Michele was growing a Most of the time she "knows" who's at the door and who's on the phone. Surprising her takes a great deal of planning and a reasonable large amount of pure treachery. I've only been successful at totally surprising her two or three times in the more that thirty-five years I've known her. It's usually a lot more work than it's worth. But not so, this time, I decided. This time I'd floor her with a surprise.

The following Friday, the guy who drove the truck across the country called and said that he was at the Framingham off ramp of the Massachusetts Turnpike. Where, he wanted to know, did he deliver the furniture?

I gave him instructions to the house, told him to get started unloading, that I'd be out in a couple of hours. I called the Real Estate guy and asked him to please go over to the house and let the movers in. Our stuff was here at last.

Next, I called the travel agent and scheduled three seats on the mid-morning flight out of Las Vegas to Boston for the girls on Monday. Then I called Patsy.

"Get to Boston. The stuff is here," I shouted with great joy.

I next rushed to clean up my desk and head out to Sudbury. The Monday morning show was all booked so I could get a head start on the weekend. It was going to be a busy two and a half days. I left BZ at twelve-thirty that Friday.

When I got to the house, the movers were trying to get the appliances up to the front door, through the snow. The narrow path that had been shoveled wasn't wide enough. I grabbed a snow shovel and started to work. By dark, we had everything out of the truck and either in the living room or in the two car garage. I signed the company voucher and the movers headed up the pike to their next stop, somewhere in sub zero Maine. I turned around and faced a mountain of boxes and cartons. (Westinghouse later said that they had "forgotten" to pay to have them unpacked.)

I had managed to get the movers to put the washer and dryer downstairs in the basement and to help me set up the beds, but that was all they would do before they left me there in "Citizen Kane's" warehouse.

I spent the next two days — and part of the next two nights — unpacking every box, hanging every picture, washing every dish and putting everything in every box away. Then I got rid of most of the boxes. The landlord stopped by on Sunday to see how I was doing. He actually gave me a hand for a couple of hours.

The Reeds, Carol and David, who lived across the street, dropped in with hot coffee and a sandwich and a warm welcome to Sudbury and Old Meadow Road. I was feeling very good about our move. But unpacking all that stuff and putting it all in it's place had nearly killed me. I finished sometime around one o'clock, Monday morning.

On Monday evening I drove through the Callahan Tunnel to Logan International Airport for a greatly anticipated rendezvous with my girls.

Working for a big TV station carries certain very nice privileges. I called the United Airlines Operations office, before I left for Logan. I told them that I was a producer with "BZ". I said that I had a special VIP guest coming in on flight 234. I requested special gate privileges. No problem, said UAL. "We're happy that your guest selected United."

In 1969, Logan Airport didn't have a covered jetway at every gate. The Boeing 727, out of Chicago where the girls had changed planes from Las Vegas, would deplane its passengers down the plane's own rear stairway, which lowered from under the tail of the airplane, onto the cold tarmac outside gate seventeen. The passengers would then have to walk the forty feet or so to the gate door and enter the terminal.

I flashed my brand new "BZ" ID at the agent and walked right through the gate, out onto the tarmac. The plane was just pulling up. The rear stair was soon deployed and I took up a position just to the side, watching for a familiar face to appear at the top of the stairs.

After a dozen or so traveling salesmen and a couple of tourists came off, I recognized two tiny blonds, carefully coming down the stairs. Teresa was holding Michele's hand, making sure she didn't slip on the cold steps. As yet, however, there was no sign of the mother of my children on those stairs.

"Hi, guys. Where's mom? She didn't get off in Chicago did she?

"Hi, Dad. No! She's coming. She doesn't move very fast these days," Charlie said with serious, seven year old worldly wisdom. "She's pregnant, you know."

"How was the flight?" I laughed as I hugged them both and got a smother of kisses in return.

"Great. But mom's real tired," Michele said.

They both looked so good to me. Michele actually looked a lot better then she had when I left her only two weeks ago in Boulder City.

"Gee, you guys look good to me. I've really missed you like crazy."

"We're sorry we lost JoJo, Dad."

"Me, too, honey."

In a couple of minutes, Patsy's head appeared at the top of the ramp. I slipped by the two people who were on the ramp, went up the stairs and took hold of her arm. She flashed me one of those great smiles, like the one that I had originally fallen in love with ten years before, and squeezed my hand.

"Welcome to Boston," I said as I handed her a brand new, warm, fur hat which I had purchased a few days earlier at Jordan Marsh, just for this occasion .

"It's very nice to be here, at last."

At the bottom of the ramp we kissed and hugged and held each other for a long, long moment. Goodness, I had missed this lady a lot. Trust me, an Angel fish just isn't the same as a wife.

"You've grown a bit in two weeks," I said as I held her away so I could look at her expansive tummy.

"I feel like a blimp. I must be twice as big as I was with the first two."

"No. You were a blimp both times then, too," I reassured her.

"I've really missed you," she said with another big grin.

"I've missed the three of you, too. Let's take your mother home, girls."

"Good idea," said Charlie.

All the way to Sudbury the girls were thrilled by the snow and the ice and the beautiful winter scene they saw flashing by outside the news car's windows. Snow was everywhere. It was in the trees, on the road, piled beside the road and on all the roofs. It was a winter wonderland to them. They had never seen snow before, except on Christmas cards or on TV.

On the way home I baited my trap. I told Patsy that I'd managed to get the beds set up and the appliances plugged in, but that the boxes were just stacked inside the house. I told her that they were mostly in the living room and the fourth bedroom. I spun my web of deceit as I told her to take her time getting them all unpacked. I'd help in the evenings, I said, but if it took us two weeks to get everything unpacked, so what? I should have been given an Academy Award for my performance that night.

When we drove up the driveway the girls couldn't believe their eyes. The house was as pretty as any Christmas Card from New England, complete with lighted, if snow covered, street side lamp post at the bottom of the driveway. All Patsy could see, however, was a warehouse stacked full of boxes, just beyond that cheery front yard. The four of us walked, very carefully, up the icy walkway, then up the four slippery steps to the front door.

I opened the door, holding back the girls so Patsy could go into her new house, first.

"Welcome home, my love," I said.

She walked through the door, took one look around, sat down on the couch and burst into tears. She couldn't believe her eyes and I couldn't believe that I had actually been able to completely surprise her!

At Logan Airport, after I was sure the plane had landed but before it had pulled up to the gate, I called my new Sudbury neighbor, Carol Reed. She and her husband, David, had gone over to the house, turned on the lights, built a fire in the fireplace, lit candles and turned on the stereo. Patsy walked into a home that was all ready to live in — everything was unpacked, hung, put away and in place. I had even gone shopping, filling the refrigerator and the pantry with food. We could have breakfast without going to the store in the morning. Patsy walked into her own home, with all her things in place, instead of a warehouse filled with boxes.

It was one of the few times I was able to completely surprise my dear wife. And this time, it was really worth the effort, believe me.

The girls, of course, took it all in stride. After all, wasn't their room supposed to be all ready for them when they arrived home from a long flight across the country?

"Mrs. Nolan, there is no easy way
to tell you what I must tell you.
The x-rays show that the cancer has returned.
"No," I cried out, "That's not possible.
You told me her kidney x-rays were all negative."

Chapter Six

First X-Rays Fine, I'll Call Later!

The next few days were spent getting Teresa enrolled in Horse Pond School, which was located just at the end of the block so she was able to cut through the woods to the school yard. We were also able to locate the best supermarket, open a bank account and meeting the neighbors. I loved Sudbury and I loved 6 Old Meadow Road.

We told our families when we left for the east that we might be there for as long as two years. As it turned out, we lived in the Boston suburb of Sudbury for eleven and a half years.

We had moved east with all of Michele's x-rays, records, files, history and notes. The records filled an entire small suitcase. Some of the x-rays were packed in with the pictures and paintings.

I had been directed by the staff at Childrens Hospital in Los Angeles to make an appointment with the clinic at something called The Jimmy Fund, within the first few weeks after we arrived in Boston.

So, when things settled down a bit, a couple of weeks after we arrived in Sudbury, I called The Jimmy Fund — today officially known as the Dana Farber Cancer Research Center — to make an appointment for Michele to have a blood study and a series of x-rays, all part of a normal follow up study for a Wilm's patient.

I was anxious to become acquainted with the doctors at The Jimmy Fund who would be following Michele's progress as she continued to improve after the surgery and recover from the first course of radiation.

The receptionists at the Jimmy Fund told us to come in on the following Monday about ten. The tests and examination would take several hours, she said.

Next, they gave me detailed instructions on how find my way through the labyrinth of streets in that section of Boston. Getting to the Jimmy Fund turned out to be quite a treasure hunt on that first visit, even with good instructions.

When we arrived at The Jimmy Fund, at that time housed in a wonderful old brick building across a small street from Childrens Hospital, we checked in at the reception desk and handed over Michele's x-rays, reports and her medical history from Los Angeles.

About 30 minutes later, a man entered the reception area and said, "Michele? Mrs. Nolan? I'm Dr. Traggis. I'll be in charge of Michele's follow up and her care here at the Jimmy Fund."

Dr. Demetrius Traggis was a small, thin, fragile, almost gaunt, man. He had a shy, gentle, quiet manner about him. I liked him almost immediately.

Over the next three years, Dr. Traggis and I would get to know each other extremely well. I grew to love and deeply respect this quiet, dedicated man of medicine.

Dr. Traggis took each of his cancer plagued children directly into his heart. I watched as the daily strain of trying to cure children from a series of terrible, life-threatening diseases — collectively known as cancer — took its terrible toll on this dedicated physician. I saw it age him and I watched as it depressed him. I knew in my heart that one day he would have to leave oncology treatment and move on to another area of clinical medicine. Cancer in children was just too hard on this wonderful man. As it is on many people in medicine.

Eventually, he did leave The Jimmy Fund. But, for the next three years, Demetrius Traggis would belong to Michele, and to me ...and we would belong to him.

On this first day at The Jimmy Fund, he sat down on a small table beside the couch where I was seated. He seemed to have no big ego nor even a hint of a medical superiority complex.

Here was an incredibly intuitive man and I could see immediately that he was able to communicate easily with people, from the very beginning, on a very personal — very comfortable — level.

"We've examined all the x-rays and the history you brought with you and now we need to take some new x-rays and conduct some new blood tests, for an updated comparison," he said with a warm touch of my hand.

"But, she looks like she's doing fine. How's she been feeling, since the trip from L.A.?"

I told him that the trip had tired us all, but that she seemed to be fine. She was eating and sleeping well and she had even gained a couple of ounces of weight in the last few weeks.

We entered the x-ray department thinking that we were just going through another diagnostic routine, just as we had several times in Los Angeles.

The first x-rays — focusing on both the original tumor area and the remaining kidney — were all clear, but there were still the chest x-rays to take before we moved on to the blood tests.

Knowing that he was very anxious to know how things were going, I called Patrick at the station to give him the good news. Patrick was not in the production office. He had gone down to the studio. I told Connie, his assistant producer, not to bother paging him or trying to transfer the call.

"Just give him a message when he comes back to the office, Connie."

"Sure!"

Connie took one of those, "While You Were Out" slips and wrote, "First x-rays, Fine. I'll Call Later!,"

When he returned from the studio, Connie handed Patrick the message, telling him that I had sounded very happy and relaxed on the phone.

In her charming, southern accented voice, she said, "I think everything's just fine."

Patrick read the message asking, "Is that all she said?"

"She said she'd call as soon as the chest x-rays were done, before she headed for home. Everything sounded very good," Connie told him again.

Patrick stuck the message in his permanent, personal telephone book (he carried that message in his phone book for at least 15 years) and continued with his preparations for the new show, feeling slightly little less worried about Michele.

A few minutes after they had taken the chest x-rays, Dr. Traggis came out to the waiting area and asked me to come back into his office with him.

He said, "Mrs. Nolan, there is no easy way to tell you what I must tell you. The x-rays show that the cancer has returned."

"No!" I cried out, "That's not possible, you said her kidney x-rays were all negative."

"Yes, her kidney x-rays look fine, but there is now clear evidence that the cancer is present in both of her lungs. I have the x-rays here, so I can show you what I mean. There's no tumor, but what you can see are these scattered spots of the disease. It's worse in the left lung, for some reason, but it's at a very early stage. Very early. And that, as you know, is a very good sign."

"Good sign?" I thought. "Good sign? What the hell does he mean, good sign?"

As I looked at those grotesque black and white pictures, I started to cry. It was so damn unfair. We had done all the things we were supposed to do, yet it was still in her body.

"What do we do now?" I asked through the tears.

"We begin chemotherapy and radiation therapy today, but I think we should also talk to Dr. Robert Filler. He's our chief of surgery. He'll probably suggest that we do an exploratory operation to see if the tumor has returned to the original tumor site or, what could potentially be much worse, to see if the disease has attacked Michele's remaining kidney. You did say she has had some slight abdominal pains over the past several weeks, didn't you?"

My world was closing back in and getting black again. Now, I had to go tell Patrick that our daughter was still infected with this terrible cancer that seemed to be playing with us. I didn't want to call him with this news. I had to touch him and I wanted his arms around me. I was scared to death all over again.

I took Michele and drove to the studios of WBZ-TV. I hated walking through those doors. I hated bringing Patrick the news I had to bring him.

Connie and I were hip deep in a dozen things to do with the new show when the door to our windowless office on the mezzanine level of the broadcast complex cracked opened a few inches and I saw the tiny, drawn face of Michele peek around the edge. It was followed by Patsy's ashen face. Pats was carrying Michele and her eyes told me that something terrible was the matter.

"What's wrong? I thought you were going to call," I said pushing her back out into the hallway where we could have some privacy from the production staff that was overflowing the small production office.

"Oh, Patrick. It's back!"

She put her free arm around my neck and sobbed into my shoulder. My heart sank through the floor.

"Back? Back where? How? What?"

"It's in her lungs. That damn stuff is in both of her lungs. They think it might be in the other kidney, too."

I uttered a soft expletive, under my breath. We just stood there, the three of us holding on to each other. What the hell were we going to do now?

About that time, a young fellow who had just been promoted to staff announcer came down the hall. He was one of the first people to make me feel welcome during my very first day on the job, a little over three weeks ago.

Charlie Austin stopped and put his arms around the three of us.

"What's up?" Charlie asked.

"The cancer's back. It's in her lungs now, Charlie."

"Damn," was all he said.

We just stood there for a few minutes, two scared people and one sick little girl being held in the strong arms of a big, warm, wonderful — near stranger — who seemed, somehow, to share our desperate pain. As I write this, I've loved Charlie Austin for over twenty-five years, but never more than I did at that moment in the hallway of WBZ in Boston as he held us in his arms and shared our pain.

"What now?" I asked.

"Well, they want to operate again and see if it's in her other kidney."

"Can't they tell that with the tests?" I wondered.

"If they wait for it to show up in a test it'll be too late for Michele, honey. We'll lose the other kidney and she'll really be in trouble. We might actually lose her, if that happens. They say that the most aggressive thing is usually the best thing with Wilm's.

"They want to schedule the operation for Monday morning. The sooner the better with this type of cancer, they say. It grows so damn fast."

"Who does the operation? I don't want any more Morton Woolleys," I reminded her — flashing back to those terrible experiences with the surgeon at Childrens in Los Angeles.

"Neither do I, believe me. You know that. But I've just come from a visit with Bob Filler. He's The Chief of Pediatric Surgery at Childrens Hospital. The Jimmy Fund is associated with Childrens. You don't even have to go outside to get from one building to the other. You just walk across a bridge.

"Honey, he spent a long time talking to me, explaining what he felt needed to be done and done quickly. Bob Filler is as far from Woolley as one can be and still be from the planet earth. He's really a very nice guy who speaks English and who seems to be our kind of doctor."

"He'd better be, if he knows what's good for him," I said.

I wasn't about to be left in the waiting room again while some egotistical surgeon found himself too busy to keep us in the loop.

As it turned out, Robert Filler, M.D. was all that we could have possible hoped for, and much, much more. That's just one of the reasons he is one of the people to whom we have dedicated this book. Without Bob Filler, there would be no book and probably no Michele.

We might note here that twenty years later, in 1989, just after we moved to Whidbey Island here in Washington, Michele developed a constriction of her bowel — as a result of the massive radiation she received as a child. The first thing I did was call Bob Filler, now the Chief of Pediatric Surgery at The Hospital for Sick Children in Toronto, Canada. Bob called one of his former students, Dr. David Tapper, Chief of Surgery at Childrens in Seattle. Dr. Tapper called me as soon as he finished talking to Bob. As we were discussing Michele's current problem, I told David Tapper that he sounded a lot like a clone of Bob Filler.

"I should," he said. "He trained me."

Dr. Tapper, who, of course, like Bob, doesn't treat adults, called his friend and colleague, John Ryan, M.D., who also trained in Boston, at Massachusetts General Hospital.

"Ryan didn't train with us over at the Brigham, he was at Mass General. But he worked under a really terrific surgeon at Mass General. A guy named, George Nardi.

"David," I said, "Dr. Nardi took out my appendix and Patsy's gall bladder. It sure is a very small medical world out there."

George Nardi was one of my heroes. I was sure that John Ryan was going to be just great for Michele.

Four days later, Michele had a gastric reconstruction to bypass the constriction in her bowel. She was a guest at Virginia Mason Hospital in October of 1989.

But, twenty years before that, in Boston, while standing in the hallway of WBZ-TV after hearing the news that we weren't yet out of the woods with this killer, that terrible fear again burned in my stomach and clutched at my throat. Here I was, just beginning to relax and feel that the awful nightmare was over, when it roared back into our lives and into Michele's tiny body. In my stomach there was such a searing pain it felt like I had swallowed a huge hot rock. That pain tore at the lining of my stomach with its sharp claws. I can only tell you that it was a white hot pain of sheer terror.

The pain and fear I saw that day on Patsy's face, just doubled my own. My beautiful little baby girl was being attacked by a bitter foe and my wonderful wife and partner was in the pain that only the mother of a sick child can experience. While I loved Michele with all my heart, I had not carried her in my womb for nine months. I had not welcomed the contractions, strain and pain that brought Michele into the world. I was her parent, but Patsy was her mother and Michele's mother was hurting like hell. I didn't know what to do about it. Plus, I was scared to death myself, all over again. It was sure a good thing that we had each other at that moment.

But, this wasn't a time to sit down and give up. There were things which had to be done. I asked Patsy if she was able to drive home. She said she was okay. I kissed them both goodbye and sent them on home.

I told Pats that I was going to make a few phone calls on BZs phone bill. I'd be along, soon.

First, I called my Mom and told her that we needed her to come to Boston, now, if she could. She, of course, was horrified that Michele was ill again, but said she'd come immediately, of course.

I'd already arranged for a ticket to be waiting for her at the American Airlines counter at LAX. I told her to plan to be with us for a while, but I didn't know just how long we would need her to stay. We wouldn't know what we were really facing until after the surgery. Crying when we hung up, she said she would see me tomorrow night, in Boston.

Now, my Mom is not the most courageous person who's ever lived. She's afraid of lots of things, including flying. Although she has done quite a bit of flying, she's never comfortable in the air. Now, here I was, asking her to drop everything and fly off across the country, alone, and give us a hand with the family while we faced yet another battle with this slick, crafty, wicked disease that had been quietly hiding there somewhere in that tiny body of Michele's for the last four months.

After I told the brass at the station what was happening and finished my calls, I got really mad. For the first time, I got really angry at the disease itself. It had been lying to the blood tests, lying to the x-rays and lying to the doctors. We thought we'd licked it, kicked it out, but, as we were to discover, this frightening malignancy would not go quietly into that dark night of oblivion. It was back and, once again, I was scared to death it might win. I was also damn mad.

Believe me, the panic you feel is not eased because you've been through it before. The thought that this deadly disease — cancer — had once again reached out and attacked a small, defenseless, helpless child is hard to even imagine. The realization that it was actually happening, nearly froze me with terror — again. But this time there was an added dimension — I was mad at the disease, at the cancer, at the invader. I wanted to reach in and rip it's head off.

"You bastard, come out and fight. Fight me. Just leave my kid the hell alone. If you're so tough, take me on, if you dare. Just get the hell away from Michele," I screamed in the Mustang on my way home as tears ran down my face and blurred my vision. I hated that cancer. I hated it with all my might. I was determined that it would not win.

Tiny and innocent, Michele had bravely dealt with her first surgery. She had held up valiantly to the terrible effects of the radiation treatments and she had been so brave for someone so young and so seriously ill. She had complained only when something was painful. She had endured the awful vomiting that the radiation brings on, without much more than a whimper. Here was one of the bravest people I have ever known, being asked, at the tender age of three, to take up the sword and do battle with this deadly, formidable foe, once more. We were asking a baby to go up against the real bogey man. A bogey man who carried a lethal bite.

I was mad as hell at the "thing" that was growing in her, but there was no way I could step in and take her place. And I gladly would have taken her place, just as any parent would when something — anything — bad happens to a child. That seems to be the one universal reaction everyone has when a child is taken seriously ill: "Take me, instead. Leave my child alone" says every parent.

I screamed out loud at that damn disease.

"Why did you have to attack my little girl, you bastard?"

"Why not attack a murderer or a child molester? Why my little girl? Why not me?"

But it does not, it seems, work that way. Our tiniest, most vulnerable member was the one being asked to do battle with this dreaded, terrifying enemy. All a parent can do at a time like this is stand by and hope you make the right decisions about the weapons.

If you should find yourself in that spot, act. Don't let the situation overwhelm you or cause you to freeze up. The best chance your child has for survival is to have you join the fight with all your guns blazing.

You can have a major effect on the outcome because you select the care, the doctors and the direction which that care will take. The burden to make those decisions wisely and make them well, is an awesome burden for any parent. There is so much room for error on this unfamiliar ground. There are so many unknowns, so many variables. Nothing can completely prepare you for this obligation, but you must take charge.

First, you dare not trust the medical world completely — their judgment is, after all, not without flaws.

Yet you must depend on the medical establishment, too, to provide some important troops to aid in your child's fight for life. Selecting the correct warriors and their weapons, I believe, is the real trick to success.

You must never doubt your ability to make the correct choices, however. You are the one your child is depending on for survival. I found that when I was the patient, these choices were actually a lot easier to make. After all, I was making decisions about my own life. But when the patient is your child, the pressure and the responsibilities for making the right choices are multiplied and compounded tenfold. You're completely responsible for that little child. Do not shrink from that responsibility. You accepted that responsibility when you elected to become this child's parent. If you ever find yourself in that unenviable position, you must live up to that responsibility.

And somehow, you will. I didn't think I could do it, but somehow I did. Exercising that responsibility became the difference between life and death, in our case. Without our active participation in the process, Michele would have surely died in Boston, as a four year old child.

While Woolley, in looking back, had not been such a poor choice as a surgeon, he had been a dreadful choice as a physician. He was a reasonably skilled, highly educated, egotistical mechanic, but not a sensitive, caring healer. The decision to move to Boston had been a calculated risk and it was, at least when we first arrived there, hard to say whether that decision had been a wise one or a poor one.

The selection of a new surgeon would also affect how the decision to move clear across the country with a cancer patient will be viewed by history. If we lost Michele in Boston would our family and friends second guess us and say that she might have lived, had we stayed the course in Los Angeles? These were not easy times for a scared parent.

The next day, Tuesday, turned out to be one of the most critical days for all of us in this adventure with Michele and her cancer.

As I sat there at work, behind my new desk, in this new job, in this new city, pondering this new phase of Michele's illness, I made an important decision. As it turned out it was a very vital decision for Michele.

I decided that Pats and I would, beginning today, take a leading part in this battle. We were no longer going to just sit on the sidelines, letting events wash over us, hoping for the best, much as we had in Los Angeles.

From now on, I promised myself, we were going to have a voice — sometimes a loud, shattering voice — in all of the upcoming medical events relating to Michele's health and treatment. From this day on, we were going to be active players in this drama — not just spectators wringing our hands on the sidelines.

From that day to this, when it comes to any medical aspect of my family's life, I have insisted that Pats and I be an integral part of the medical team. As you might imagine, that is not always a popular position with many of those involved, either in the practice of medicine or in the delivery of health care services. But it's a decision which I have never withdrawn from — the bitter, often harsh, criticism of others aside — nor is it one I have ever regretted.

The decision to be informed, interactive participants in the health care of our family has always held us in good stead. While not all of our decisions have been perfect, we do have a very, very high batting average. And you will too. Follow your heart, but be guided by your head.

Our success has been high because we both made the decision to be informed players, not just nervous watchers. We insist on being told the facts — even when one of the things we learn from the doctors may simply be, "At this point, we just don't know."

Most of the medical world has lost sight of the fact that they work for the rest of us. We — or our insurance companies — hire them to do what we are unable to do for ourselves. But that doesn't mean we stop thinking or reasoning for ourselves.

And it never means that we hand our child to some "highly regarded" M.D. and leave the room, hoping that this fine representative of of the medical world will do the right thing. When you take your car to the mechanic you want to know what's wrong, what he thinks needs to be done and how he plans to do it. Many times we want to see the broken part or the worn component that needs replacing or repair. Why should we give any broader license to a person whose name is followed by the initials M.D.?

Particularly when that person is going to treat our child.

Of course, Pats and I recognize that there are some people who do not want to know every little detail about what the medical team does to them — or to a member of their family. But we should all be active partners in the treatment of an illness which invades our lives or the lives of our loved ones, even when it's not comfortable for us to do so. We must insist on being full partners in the healing effort.

It is only now, with the shouts and screams of a few of us ringing in their ears, that the medical community — doctors mostly — are starting to discover that a team approach to the problem enjoys greater results than would be achieved if the care had been purely clinically professional.

The doctor, who once wanted to be the great god-like figure who did all the talking, gave all the instructions and made all the decisions, is giving way to the doctor of the twenty-first century who understands that with the informed support of the family — or even that of the patient's close friends — positive results for the patient can be absolutely, and sometimes astonishing, improved.

But in 1969, except for a few enlightened and confident doctors such as Demetrius Traggis and Bob Filler, the doctors of the world were still trying to pat our hands and tell us, "Please don't worry. Everything's going to be just fine. We'll take care of it."

Some doctors still try to withhold every drop of information, thinking that we are either too dumb to comprehend what it is they would tell us, or that we're too scared to even want to hear it. Both excuses are, of course, almost always completely invalid.

I believe that there's more to their manufactured aura of mystery than just the judgment that we're too uneducated — medically, or too scared of what we'll hear. I believe there's a fear, on the part of a lot of medical folks, that to let us behind that curtain — like the curtain in "The Wizard of Oz" — it will reveal the terrible truth about medicine and medical people.

Many of them are terrified that we will learn that they have no magic, no special secrets, no special powers. I think they are afraid that we'll see the simple truth.

The truth which many of them are terrified that we will discover is that they are highly trained, well educated, supremely skilled, vastly experienced and, in many cases, extremely gifted and special people — who have no special, magic power. They, just like the rest of us, are only mere mortals, earning a living.

Those scardy cats are actually doing their patients a great disservice when they shrink behind their name badges, lab coats, special language and their superior, aloof and arrogant attitudes. Healing is stifled when they try to treat us from on high.

If, on the other hand, they let their patients — and their patient's families — become partners in their own health care, a dramatically improved level of healing is almost always realized. Fears — in both the patients and in the families — are lessened. Tensions between the medical world and the rest of us mere mortals are reduced. Recovery is more rapid. Plainly put: people get better faster.

But when the medical folks decide to withhold information, act in secrecy, or deal with us as though we're too uneducated to comprehend either what they do or what they think is wrong with us, they allow our imaginations to run wild — crazy with fear and tormented with misunderstanding.

Most of us are too timid — as I had been during my three encounters with Woolley — and too cowardly to say, "Hold it, just a second. I want to know what you know and I want to know what you don't know about my child and her illness. And I want to know right now. Not when you find the time in your busy schedule to tell me, but right now, please."

Face it. Doctors scare the hell out of most of us. We're afraid to ask them anything, much less challenge or confront them when we feel they are not treating us the way we think we should be treated.

Many doctors — and even a lot of paramedics and a few nurses — have carefully developed the attitude of being above the rest of us — unassailable. Although I am happy to say that, like the Berlin Wall, that attitude is beginning to crumble. But bring your "attitude hammer" to the next encounter you have with a doctor. If he walls himself up behind his title — "Call me, Doctor Jones, Bill" — and doesn't agree to make you a partner in your own health care or fails to give you full and complete answers which you can understand, take out your hammer and take a few chips off the wall. If you don't see a change in that attitude, get up and walk out.

Most medical doctors are trained to be superior and unequal. The first symptom of this attitude is the insistence that even in the most intimate moment — a moment when we may be discussing life and death — that we still address them in a very formal manner. Have you ever noticed that only the really good physicians ask people to call them by a real name? Most of them expect us to call all of them by the very same first name, Doctor. A young doctor — even just a graduate, with the ink still fresh on his M.D. certificate — can call a ninety-seven year old lady Sara, but he still wants her to address him as, Doctor Jones. It's all part of the mystic of being a doctor, with that carefully orchestrated atmosphere of control.

Don't fall for it for even one more day. The next time you have an occasion to talk with a doctor you know, any doctor — even your dentist — call him Bob (or whatever his name actually happens to be). My dentist, has lowered himself to the level of allowing his patients to call him, Doctor Mark. Right! He calls me Patrick. I call him Mark.

Think of this. Medical doctors, and to some degree dentists too, expect to be addressed by their educational credentials. Wouldn't it sound a little silly to run around calling people, Bachelor Bob or Masters Eddie? People would think you'd either been a contestant on the dating game or that you play a great game of chess or bridge.

That, "Call me, Doctor Jones," business is just another barrier the medical world has constructed in the path of getting the best possible medical care. And, while I'm on the subject, never forget where the buck actually stops.

Never forget — when we're talking about this medical team — that you, as the patient — if you're an adult — or as the parent, if the patient is your child, are the head of the team. The doctors, nurses and technicians are just advisors, workers and practitioners. They explain to you the options, while you, as the team leader, make the informed decisions about what course the treatment will take. But, without information, how can you possibly make an informed decision?

The answer is, of course, you can't!

Information is power. If the doctor withholds vital information, he's in control. If you have that information, you can control the direction of things and take an active role in bringing about the best possible outcome.

So whatever it takes — screaming, hollering, threatening, insisting or banging your fist on the desk — get the information you need. ALL the information. Especially if that information is a doctor's clear and direct admission of: "I don't know what's wrong."

Always remember, it's perfectly all right for a doctor not to know what's wrong, but it sure as hell isn't all right for her to pretend she does know, when actually she doesn't.

I have much more respect for a medical care provider who says, "I don't know!" then I have for the ones who try to avoid the question or "snow" me with medical gibberish.

There are people in the medical profession who say that life and death decisions are too important to be made by the family (or even the patient). They say that these are "medical decisions," as though only those with a degree in medicine are ever capable of making a medical decision. That's just more of their controlling rhetoric. Don't let them get away with it, not even for five seconds.

There are a lot of very fine physicians, dedicated to providing the finest possible care to those in pain, in trouble and in need. There are thousands, maybe tens of thousands of Bob Fillers and Larry Pages out there practicing medicine, making people better and operating with the very best interests of the patient and the family in the forefront at all times.

But there is also a number of money mad, power crazed Docs who have built a galvanized wall around their investment portfolios. They see any reduction in their system of control as a serious threat to their position as a "supreme person."

Whenever you encounter one of these jerks, run as fast as your legs will carry you to a Robert Filler type of physician. Never look back and never feel guilty. You wouldn't feel guilty about firing your gardener if he was killing the plants or selling off your trees, would you?

Of course you wouldn't, but the gardener doesn't have the letters M.D. behind his name.

When you take firm control of the medical situation, you have just taken the first big step toward saving your child's life.

That night, when he got home, Patrick told me how strongly he felt that we must from now on assert ourselves more deeply in every aspect of Michele's care. I knew he was right, but it wouldn't be at all easy for me, at first. For me, having been trained as a nurse, being subservient to doctors was natural, was ingrained in me by the system. In school, I had been carefully taught to be a member of the, "Yes, Doctor, whatever you say" group. Although there were times when I had questioned a doctor's orders, I was always more comfortable just following their directives.

I promised Patrick that I would make every effort to take charge even though I knew he would have to be our team captain.

A couple of days later, we checked Michele into Childrens Hospital in Boston. My new resolve to be more deeply involved would soon be tested.

Patrick's Mom had arrived from California to help with the family. She was very distressed about the new surgery.

"It's just like taking a little lamb to slaughter," she said, sadly, as we posed the girls for a picture in the front yard before we left for the hospital.

She was, of course, right. It was April and spring had come to New England. It was a time of new buds and green grass and new life. Both

Patrick and I were feeling serious doubts about this impending operation. Did we really have to take this seemingly healthy, happy child back to those swinging, electric doors marked — Surgery, Keep Out?

It just didn't seem right somehow.

Was this the first place to assert our new determination to lead the medical team? Did this surgery need to be performed or was this another case of the doctors wanting to control?

We met with Bob Filler at Michele's bedside the day before the surgery. Bob said, yes, the best thing he could tell us after the operation would be that the surgery had been totally unnecessary. This exploratory "look," he explained, was only to check for any cancerous involvement in her remaining kidney. In fact, the "spots" of the disease in her lungs were already being reduced successfully by radiation, which had been started the day they were discovered.

"Today's x-ray showed a marked improvement," he said. "The spots in her lung will probably mostly be gone before we even do the operation tomorrow. But, we've got to see if there's any cancerous involvement in that other kidney. If it's been affected, we need to know before it shows up on the kidney function tests."

These were the primitive days before CAT scans and MRIs.

"We must attack this disease aggressively, if we want to keep her," Bob told us. "This type of cancer grows far too fast for us to sit and wait for it. This is a deadly game with a sneaky, deadly opponent and we need to be well ahead of it if we want to win. I have every reason to believe that we can win, but we'll need to be a little lucky tomorrow. We really want this is be a completely unneeded operation."

The next day the much dreaded, "unneeded" operation was over in just an hour and a half.

The news that the operation was over so quickly scared the hell out of Patrick.

"It must be bad news, Pats," he said flatly. "Bob must have just taken one look and closed her back up. She hasn't been up there long enough."

Patrick was really depressed, having expected a much longer day. Now, as we waited for Bob to join us, Patrick was fearing the very worst.

They have a wonderful system at Childrens in Boston. There is a nurse (on this day it was a nurse named Mrs. Overstreet) assigned just to those families whose children are in surgery. As the surgery progresses, this special nurse regularly checks to see what's happening in the OR. She always knows where the parents are, whether they're in the cafeteria, the waiting room or in the garden out back.

Another wonderful thing about Childrens Hospital in Boston is this very comfortable, cozy room, just off the lobby, where the doctor meets you right after the operation. It's a gentle, warm room, with sofas, and tables and real lamps — not ceiling fixtures of fluorescent lights and plastic benches. It's a totally private place to receive bad news and a quiet place to get the good news. It's a wonderful idea and it's leagues ahead of the sterile visitors lounge or busy hallways used for such conferences in most hospitals.

As we waited there in that room for Bob to come down from the OR, our hearts were in our throats. We just held each other's hand without talking.

Finally, after what seemed like an hour, but was actually only minutes, Bob walked through the door.

"She's fine," were the first words out of Bob's mouth.

"It went really well. There's no involvement in the left kidney at all — it's completely clear and normal. It's bigger than normal, but that's what happens when we lose one at an early age, the other one compensates by growing larger than it would if both were still present."

"I was able to remove some of the scar tissue, contusions and other things that have caused her some discomfort since the first surgery, so this wasn't a completely wasted procedure today. She should be a lot more comfortable now, after she recovers from today's action. But, in general, it looks very good. Now, how are you two doing?" he asked, touching my hand.

Bob Filler is a very kind and thoughtful and healing man, besides being a gifted surgeon.

We told him that we were really concerned when we heard that it was over so soon. We thought that might mean bad news.

"I'm sorry," he said, "I guess I didn't take enough time to explain how long I expected things to take. My fault and I'm sorry if I added to your stress."

We told him not to worry about us, we were now doing fine and that we were very thankful to be here in Boston with him and not in L.A. with another doctor. A doctor we didn't name.

In a few minutes, we were in the recovery room as the process of recovering from the trauma of surgery again began for Michele. But this time her recovery would be a little easier. The surgery hadn't been as invasive as the first time. The trauma hadn't been as deep and the damage hadn't been as extensive either. There wasn't even a new incision. Bob had just reopened a small section of the original incision.

Seeing your baby in the recovery room, just after surgery, is a very difficult experience for a mother — even a mother who's trained as a nurse. There before her is the one she's given birth to, and promised to care for and protect, wrapped in bandages, with tubes taking fluids out of her body and other tubes delivering life sustaining fluids into her body.

Michele looked so tiny laying there on that big gurney. So tiny and fragile and vulnerable. The urge to reach down and pick her up and hold her in my arms had to be overcome by practicality and reason. Once more, a mother is asked to react "reasonably," rather than emotionally. It's a very hard thing to do, but it's even harder to shield your child from any sense of your own fear or anxiety.

The baby before you is the major combatant in a struggle for life. She must be comforted and supported and encouraged, but never frightened or confused. She needs to know she's winning the struggle. Any hint in your voice or any look on your face that betrays that positive attitude can be devastating. Any reason to mistrust her care givers can destroy the fragile, delicate confidence that's so vital to a successful recovery.

Always remember, even as you stand by you child's bed, he is adrift on an alien spaceship, a prisoner in a strange and scary alien world, which he can't begin to understand.

As Patrick told a nurse who was attempting to make her own life a bit easier at Michele's expense, "She's on a spaceship surrounded by strangers who speak a foreign language. She needs the truth. She needs to be told — and retold — that everything is fine. She doesn't know what to expect. We have to provide those expectations and then we have to be sure we meet them. No surprises for her, no assumptions on your part. Communicate, even when you may think it's not necessary."

I don't remember much about that second trip to the hospital, but I do remember that I wasn't scared. I believe I wasn't scared because I wasn't worried about the unknown. Both mom & dad answered my questions without "making up" an answer or giving me an answer that didn't make sense. It's surprising how much adult can be found in a three year old when the situation is serious. And believe me, even at that young age, I could tell that something was very serious. Just looking at all those long faces and hearing those humorless conversations let me know — this was serious stuff.

I do remember always being very thirsty and never getting a drink when I wanted it. It was the one thing that really disturbed me about those operations. I never did buy those dumb excuses about being sick to my stomach. I wasn't feeling sick, I was feeling thirsty and I wanted a drink of water.

I also remember that they seemed to need to stick a needle in me an awful lot. I grew to hate those lab technicians who dashed into the room, said nothing, grabbed my arm, wrapped a tourniquet around it and then said, "Now, hold still, this is only going to hurt a little."

Wrong. When you're in the hospital everything hurts a little. It's just that their estimation of "just a little" and the perception of a three year old's "just a little" are vastly different. But I did prefer those who said it was going to hurt to those who lied. Yes, lied.

One time Dad told a head nurse that she couldn't give me a shot after she told me it wasn't going to hurt.

"I'm sorry," she protested, "but I have to give her this shot right now."

"No you don't," said Dad. "You can go out and come back and give it to her in five minutes. And when you do, tell her the truth. Tell her it's going to hurt. Tell her it's only going to hurt for just a second and that it's only going to hurt a little, but tell her that it's going to hurt."

"Well, we find it's a little easier if we don't scare them by telling them it's going to hurt," she said, trying to wiggle off the hook and go forward with the injection.

"Hold it!," Dad challenged her. "Easier? Easier for whom? Easier for you? Listen lady, I don't care how tough this job is on you. You elected to be here, she didn't. The only person I want things easier on is Michele and if you think I'm going to let you lie to her just to make giving her a shot easier on you, you've got another think coming."

"But I have to give her this injection and if you don't stop interfering with me I'll have to ask you to leave the room."

Dad, putting his face very close to hers, said very quietly, but very clearly, "The one who will leave is you, and right now. And should you decide to come back with that needle, you will tell her the truth. She's in a strange land here and the only thing she has on her side is me, her mom and the truth.

"Now, if you don't think that needle is going to hurt, I'll be happy to stick it in your butt and let you be the judge. You're the one who's going to leave this room. You're upsetting my daughter, nurse."

The nurse must have turned pale. She stormed back to the desk, called Dr. Filler to report what had happened — demanding that my dad be removed from the hospital, not just my room. As Dr. Filler told Mom, he asked the nurse if she had, indeed, told me that it wasn't going to hurt to be given an injection. When she admitted that she had told me that, Dr. Filler told her that she was wrong and that my dad was right and that the next time she gave a child an injection to tell the truth. The head nurse wasn't very pleased with my dad after that, but she was a little more aware of what kind of a physician our Dr. Filler was. She also learned that Dad wasn't going to let her title, her position or her authority get in the way of doing what was best for me.

I remember that my room had a lot of windows along one side — big windows, almost floor to ceiling. And I remember it rained a lot while I was there. I also remember a quiet, gentle lady who came in almost every day and washed the windows. And I remember all the toys and all the cards and all the letters.

At "BZ," in those days, besides the cool, young weather turk that every station had to have in those days of modern media consultants, we had a couple of aging weathermen. One had been there since the station went on the air.

This guy (I'm not going to mention his name here because he was never very helpful or cooperative during the year and more that he reported the weather on my morning show) was considered a real "local treasure." Today, he couldn't get a job in broadcast news, but he was, in those years, New England's Favorite Weatherman — even though he had no formal training or education in the science of predicting the weather. But he did, to his credit, know New England weather patterns fairly well. Move him and his tremendous ego to the Midwest and he would have been a joke.

The other old hand in the weather room, a guy named Norm, was a graduate of MIT where he was currently a professor of meteorology. He was the more scientific forecaster of the group. He was also the angriest.

One day, as Norm was preparing his forecast, he told me casually that he had had a daughter who developed cancer of the kidney several years before.

"She was seven years old when she died. That was the end of that marriage," he said calmly, without malice.

"Losing a child has that effect, you know? It either brings two people closer together, or it tears the marriage apart. In our case, our daughter's death destroyed our marriage. We each blamed the other for what happened, I guess."

"How could that happen?," I asked.

"Well, before you know what's happening, you find yourself moving away from your spouse. I don't know who moved first in our case, probably me," he said honestly. "But when that action starts, it's almost never reversed. I know couples who divorced when their child suffered a grave illness, and the kid lived. The trauma of the illness was just too much for the marriage, so the marriage died. Our marriage died loudly, soon after the funeral. It was probably weak or failing anyway, but when it's a kid with a serious illness or when a kid dies, lots of times the marriage dies, too. Ours sure did. I know that."

Norm never knew it, but he gave me an invaluable lesson in marriage relations that day. Not bad for an old weather guy who had been married at least three — and maybe four — times.

As the days and later the years, passed, I have often thought of that wonderful conversation with Norm. His analysis of what could happen to a marriage under the stress of a child's illness — indeed, what had happened to him — was addressed, as you might expect from an academician, in a clinically factual and purely educational way. I don't think he even knew he was warning me. He was just reporting life — or the effects of life — as he had observed it in his real studies of what life holds for us. I'll always be grateful to him for those sage comments. It put me on my guard. Norm may have even saved our marriage from a fate similar to his own. Thanks, Norm.

I have come to believe more and more over the years that Norm was absolutely right. You either came closer as husband and wife or move toward the dissolution of the marriage under the stressful circumstances involving the death or serious illness of a child. I knew which one I wanted to happen to us.

In the next few weeks, Patsy and I spent a lot of time talking about my discussion with Norm and about how we wanted to be strengthened by what was happening to Michele and not destroyed by it. We have continued, for over twenty years now, to direct our marriage in that way.

In only a few days, Michele was ready to return to Sudbury from the hospital. She was weak and a bit thinner, but she was not depressed by the surgery or the treatments. She was anxious to get on with being a little girl. She wanted to play with her sister Teresa, her new friends, Sherry and Laurie Reed, but mostly, she wanted to sleep in her very own bed. She also was anxiously waiting for the new baby. When her new brother or sister arrived, she knew she would no longer be the baby of the family.

Within a few weeks, we were even able to take her and Patrick's Mom to Maine for a typical New England clam bake outing. It turned out to be a lovely summer day on Casco Bay. I've never forgotten that marvelous clam bake on the beach.

In a few more weeks, Michele seemed to be getting completely back to normal. Patrick's Mom, who had made such heroic efforts while she was with us, was finally able to return to her home in California. Our new baby was about to join us, Patrick's morning show was doing well and the New England spring was sunny and warm. The future, again, looked bright and hopeful.

Then, just as Michele came back into the waiting room,
a man looked up and said,
"We're very fortunate that my daughter
only needs to come back here just once each year."
"You see," he said, "we live in Tel Aviv."

Chapter Seven

Those Damn Spots!

As the New England summer of 1969 came into its full, glorious bloom, our schedules became rather hectic. Patrick's new show required that he leave Sudbury before six each morning and return to us after seven most evenings. As a result, the children didn't see much of their father, until the weekend. I was busy caring for the girls, keeping the house, looking after Patrick and preparing for our new arrival who was scheduled to join us sometime during the last week in June.

I was also loading Michele into the car every morning and driving the twenty-two miles to The Jimmy Fund for her daily radiation and chemotherapy treatments. After just a few weeks, those trips became routine, but I never looked forward to them.

While the majority of the spots in Michele's lung had vanished under the beam of radiation before the last surgery, there was one collection of cancer cells which seemed particularly resistant to the treatment. That damn spot just would not go away.

The radiation therapy cycle meant that a treatment would be given five days a week for six weeks. Because there was still a spot on her left lung at the end of the first series another two week series was given, this time over just the individual spot, and not the entire lung.

The effects of radiation vary from patient to patient and Michele seemed to be uniquely able to tolerate the impact of the treatments on her system. But as the deadly beams of radiation did their work on the cancer cells, she did experience a severe loss of appetite and a feeling of fatigue and lethargy. Luckily the nausea and vomiting which commonly accompanies extensive radiation was not a serious problem for her, although there were days when she would lose what little she ate.

The radiation therapy didn't cause near the havoc that the chemotherapy did. She would receive an injection every day for seven days and then 6 weeks later she would begin again.

For about four weeks after the last injection she would be pale and tired. The last two weeks she would begin to look better. She would feel like eating full meals and she would play with the other children more and then, whammo! It was time to start the cycle all over again.

Each morning we would drive 45 minutes to the Jimmy Fund and as we drove home, Michele would generally lay quietly on the back seat of the car and doze.

One day, near the end of one of these tiresome cycles, I was feeling particularly sorry for myself.

As I sat in the waiting room while Michele received her treatment, I casually remarked to another mother there that I was really becoming tired out, having to drive so far each day.

The lady said she understood just how I felt, because she and her daughter lived in Vermont and had to come down for the entire week and stay in a boarding house near the hospital. (Unfortunately, there were no Ronald McDonald Houses back in those days.)

Another woman who was sitting just across from me in the waiting room said she was pleased that her daughter only had to come back for monthly visits. She told me that they lived in Hershey, PA, more than a full day's drive for them.

Maybe, I thought, I didn't have so much to complain about with my forty-five minute commute.

Just as Michele came back into the waiting room, a man looked up and said, "I'm very fortunate that my daughter only needs to come back to the Jimmy Fund just once each year. You see, we live in Tel Aviv."

I felt of wave of guilt sweep over my bones as he spoke. What in the world was I complaining about with my short drive through the beautiful New England countryside?

I didn't have to fly halfway around the world, transferring in London and traveling through seven time zones.

I stopped feeling sorry for myself in a big hurry, grateful that we had been fortunate enough to have moved to Sudbury, only 23 miles from The Jimmy Fund. I guess it's just a matter of perspective. None of the people in that waiting room considered their journey to be long or bothersome nor even tiresome. Each of those parents was happy to be able to bring their youngsters back to Boston. More than that, they were deeply grateful for the efforts of The Jimmy Fund which, of course, had enabled them to still have a youngster to bring back to Boston.

As long as we live, Patrick and I will always be deeply grateful to The Jimmy Fund and the wonderful staff of dedicated and skilled people who worked there during Michele's illness.

One night, after an extremely difficult day for Pats in Boston, which had included a treatment for Michele followed by a visit to a new obstetrician, she asked me a rather surprising question.

"Honey, what would you think if we decided to have this baby at home, and didn't bother with all the hospital nonsense we'll have to put up with in Boston?"

"Fine with me, but who are you going to get to come out to the house?"

She rolled laboriously over onto one side, propped her head up on an elbow and said, "I wasn't thinking about trying to tackle that assignment. What I mean is, what would you think about our just doing this thing ourselves, you and me. You've been saying all along that you wanted to do as much as the doctor would let you. Now, I'm thinking, maybe we should just forget about the hospital and their rules and regulations and have this kid, right here, in this bed, here at home."

My heart leaped with excitement, but I had to make sure she was suggesting this for the right reasons.

"Why are you bringing this up? Because you think I'll raise too much hell at the hospital when I have to fight the old delivery room battle with them all over again?," I asked.

"Partly, yes, I'll have to admit. There's only one hospital in Boston that will even agree to have you in the labor room with me, much less the delivery room. I'm just not up to another battle royal with those people, honey. But more than that, I'm not sure I can spend four days away from Michele, which is how long the doctor is saying he wants me to spend in the hospital after the birth."

There was always the thought in the back of Pats' mind that one of those days she was "resting up" in the maternity hospital could be Michele's last day anywhere.

"The guy seems like a nice enough fellow, and Boston seems to be a great place to be sick, but, my God, are the people around here in the dark ages when it comes to having babies!," she said.

"Maybe we should have stayed in L.A. instead of coming clear back here to Boston. We could have just had the baby at Ed's," I offered.

"No! The Jimmy Fund is the best place in the world for Michele. We both know that. It's just that now I'm going to have to deal with a sick child and her care and a new child and its needs. I just don't think I can handle all that's going to be involved here, if we're spread out all over town. I'd like to make it as simple as possible for you, me and both the kids.

"So," she said with that sassy smile, "just how comfortable do you feel about being a midwife, mister?"

The Walter Mitty in me was cheering. I was dancing on the ceiling. Was she kidding? I had wanted desperately to be a major player in the arrival of this new child, but it was beginning to appear as though I'd have to go to war, again, just to watch from the delivery room doorway. It was beyond my wildest dreams to have Pats suggest that we do it alone, at home. Inside, I was standing at home plate, ready to hit the home run that would win the World Series, but outwardly, I tried my best to stay calm, but I wanted to sing.

"I feel just fine about it, but what are we going to do about prenatal care for you and the baby? We want to continue to make sure that everything is okay with you and the baby, don't we?"

As usual she was way ahead of me. "I've got the name of a young OBGYN guy over in Framingham (the next town south of Sudbury) who's supposed to be progressive and enlightened and all that. I've made an appointment for Tuesday."

"I'll go with you," I said.

"No, that's not necessary. I'll just tell him that we're having the baby at home and ask him if he wants to do the prenatal exams. If he doesn't, I'll get another referral and we'll find someone else."

"Okay, but tell this guy that we don't want any medical slight of hand at the end. I don't want to get all primed to deliver my own kid at home, only to have some damn doctor decide at the last minute that he wants his fee so he tells us that he thinks that there's some vague reason why we should suddenly be in the hospital. You know, telling us that having the baby at home would be against medical advice, just so he can take charge and take control."

"I'll make it clear to him that he's got to be completely honest and up front with us. I'm sure there won't be any problem. He might decide not to become involved. Who knows?"

She was very casual about the whole thing. I was sure that she had thought the whole thing through. We were going to have this baby at home. I was going to deliver my own child. Dreams do come true. I was ecstatic. I didn't go to sleep for hours as I went over every detail of Michele's birth in my head. Walter Mitty was going to deliver his own baby. I wanted to go up on the roof and scream the news across the house tops of New England.

A few days later, when I got home from the studio, she told me that the appointment with the OBGYN that day had gone really well.

"At first, he said he didn't know if he could approve of our having the baby at home, without medical assistance," she said.

"What did you say?"

"I told him that we weren't asking for his permission. We simply wanted to know if he was interested in being paid to examine me and the baby during these last few weeks before the birth. I told him we had decided to have this child at home and we just wanted some good prenatal care, period. If he wasn't interested, we'd find someone who was. I also told him that we would not tolerate any suggestion that we have the baby in the hospital unless he had some serious and documentable evidence that it was absolutely necessary for either me or the baby to be in the hospital."

"Maybe he'll come up with some indication of trouble that he says is not provable, but that he's sure of, with his training and experience and all. You know, the old, 'Trust me,' nonsense," I suggested.

Patsy fixed me with a firm gaze. "I made our position very clear, honey. He knows that we trust only a very few doctors and that anything negative that he might tell us, anything that would make us change our plans and check into the hospital, would be viewed with serious suspicion. I told him if he did suggest that there was some medical reason why we should be in the hospital, I would not hesitate to seek a second, or even a third opinion."

"He knows how healthy I am, and have been. I reminded him that I had already experienced two previous uneventful pregnancies. I also told him that my mother had had seven completely normal pregnancies, the bulk of which were very close together, so, historically, I knew I was a prime candidate for a perfectly normal delivery. I'm sure he understands. He doesn't want to give up control, but he knows we'll walk right out if he tries to be cute with us," she said, closing the matter.

I was very, very proud of her. Given her training, this tough stance with a new doctor — one on one — had not been an easy thing for her to do. The doctor had, of course, under Patsy's conditions, agreed to be the prenatal doctor for her pregnancy.

Speaking of conditions, Pats had just one condition for me when it came to the day of the actual delivery of this child.

"Now listen to me, Mister Midwife, and listen to me very carefully. I'm having no part of cleaning up the mess after this baby's born. You do clearly understand that, don't you?"

"Sure. That's no big problem. Remember, I was there when we had Michele," I said with complete confidence.

"Patrick, the hospital delivery room and our bedroom are light years apart when it comes to managing the mess of child birth. Having a baby is a very messy business, a *very* messy business and I'm not cleaning up any of it. That's your job, period. My job is to have this monster. Your job is to clean up the mess," she said firmly.

I, of course, instantly agreed to her only condition. Who among us would be foolish enough to argue with a woman who had grown into something roughly the size of a small water buffalo?

Now, out there somewhere there may have been some people who would have been brave enough too argue the point with her, but I certainly was not among them.

We went on to discuss the fact that we would have to prepare for this blessed event. We'd need a rubber sheet for the bed, a large supply of absorbent materials and the other things that you need when babies are born. I was getting very excited. Patsy was just getting very large.

On June seventh, Michele celebrated her fourth birthday. She was feeling completely recovered from the effects of the last surgery and her appetite was returning as the radiation treatments had been halted for two weeks. She was on a schedule of once a day for ten days and then a two week rest to let her body and the normal cells recover from the radiation. The skin on her stomach and back started to thin out, developing, as her lower abdomen had during the early treatments, the appearance of finely tanned leather.

By now, after all she'd been through, Michele was, of course, just skin and bones. Had she been given a body fat test it would have been zero or certainly near zero, I'm sure. We were doing our best to get some weight back on her, but the job of fattening up Michele in those days wasn't one of the world's most rewarding occupations.

It did seem that Michele had recovered much quicker from this surgery than she had from the first one. I know that the first one was more extensive and involved a lot more internal parts, but major surgery, even through the same opening as last time, is still major surgery.

She liked to take a long nap each day after lunch. Teresa and the other members of the Old Meadow Road gang would dash off into the woods and Michele would slowly walk down the hall and crawl up on her bed with a stuffed animal and fall into a sound sleep. She could choose from about two hundred stuffed animals that were sitting on every available inch of space in her room. When grownups are sick, people send flowers. When little people are sick, they send balloons, flowers and lots and lots of stuffed animals.

As the weeks slowly dragged by, I grew increasingly weary of the growing load I was carrying and the daily routine of traveling back and forth to Boston with Michele. The month of May seemed to be eight weeks long and June moved even slower across the calendar. I didn't think this pregnancy was ever going to end.

About the middle of June, I was nearing the end of my endurance. I had gone from facing life week to week, to facing it day to day. I wasn't far from being reduced to only having an hourly perspective on my life.

June twentieth that year was our tenth wedding anniversary. Patrick planned to prepare a quiet dinner at home for the four of us. More than that was out of the question. My dancing days seemed to be lost in the mists of the past or far, far into the future. The distance, in either direction, was just too enormous to even consider.

Before dawn that morning, as he did five days a week, Patrick kissed me goodbye and left for the studio to do his show, "New England Today." He did remember to wish me a happy wedding day on his way out the door.

"Remember, I'll get everything for dinner on the way home. Happy Anniversary, Love. I'm very glad that you married me, although I don't think I'd have married you if I'd known you were going to grow to be the size of a great beached whale," he teased.

With mock homicidal effort, I threw a pillow almost half way across the room at him. He laughed and left for work.

A few hours later, I got Teresa off to school before loading Michele into the car for the forty-five minute drive to the Jimmy Fund.

I was not looking forward to this visit. Today was going to be an extra long day because Michele was scheduled for a routine series of diagnostic tests, as well as the radiation treatment. We would be sitting for long periods of time, waiting for our turn in the lab and for our turn in x-ray. By now I couldn't sit comfortably, anywhere, for more than twenty seconds. God, I wanted this child to be born.

The drive alone almost broke my poor, weary back, to say nothing of testing the absolute endurance of my bladder, an organ which, most of the time, seemed to be carrying the entire weight of the monstrous child which continued to grow — and sleep — in my womb.

Sitting for hours on those hard, plastic bucket seats that Childrens Hospital called "chairs" was pure torture, too. I can't tell you how tired I was of being pregnant. I knew the other two pregnancies couldn't have taken this long to complete. I must be getting old, I thought.

This pregnancy had been extremely long and tiresome for me. I had gotten pregnant just before Michele got sick. Then, five months into the pregnancy we had moved clear across the country, to a place where I had no friends, no family and, except for Patrick, no support system at all. I had the bulk of the burden of Michele's cancer treatment, the stress of her second surgery, the daily trips to Boston and the growing baby I was struggling to carry and keep. I'll never know why my body, under all that stress, hadn't simply rejected this baby somewhere along the way. I'm very happy that it didn't, but as I neared the end of term, I knew without a shadow of a doubt that I was more than ready to deliver this child into the world.

I had a really great gang of people working with me on the morning show that year at BZ. Connie was from Texas, accent and all, and John had graduated from Notre Dame.

In 1969, it was a rivalry made in heaven. "Hook 'em Horns" and "Fight, Fight for Old Notre Dame" were their daily battle cries. Later that year, Texas would win the big game between them on New Year's Day. Of course, when that happened, there was no living with Connie for weeks.

Wendell Davis, one of the sweetest people on the planet Earth, was our devoted on-air director. Wendy Davis was a "fixture" at WBZ. He went to work there right after college. When World War II broke out he was trooped off to serve his country, in the Navy. Wendy distinguished himself in the war, as did a dozen or so of the other employees of WBZ. Behind the door in the front lobby there's a plaque honoring the BZ employees who served in that war. Most of them are gone now, but Wendy Davis is still sailing forward on fresh winds.

I've made a real effort to stay in touch with Wendy and Anne, his lovely bride of fifty odd years, since those days at BZ. The Davises, like a lot of other folks, eventually retired and moved to Florida — partly to be near their kids, but mostly so that Wendy could sail all year long.

Wendy and Anne were both wonderful folks, more deeply in love with each other after fifty years of marriage than they were the day they married. Their love for each other was a very rare, very special thing to see.

Just knowing Wendy and his Anne, and seeing how a marriage was supposed to work — even after twenty-five years — showed Patsy and me that you could be as openly and completely in love with each other for the entire duration of your marriage as you were on the day you said "I do!"

Wendy, being a saltwater sailor (I think his blood is actually a little more salty than seawater), talked and lived with the vernacular of the sea.

There is — or at least so says Wendy — an old sailor's code between shore-bound lovers and their sea-going sailors, that when flashed ship to the shore reads only: "1 — 4 — 3."

One, four, three, a simple but eloquent code of affection. One, four, three, of course, stands for the number of letters in the age old phrase, I Love You. One, four, three. Wendy used to write little notes to Anne and, at the bottom he would write 1-4-3.

I have never known a fellow more in love than Wendy Davis was with Anne and I have also never known a more patient, kind and more in love with her guy, lady — for Anne Davis was in every good sense of the word a lady — than Anne Davis.

Only when you have made the total commitment that Anne and Wendy willingly made to each other can two people truly consider themselves to be married. Few people, even if married for half a century, ever reach that level of pure love, absolute trust and total bonding. Wendy and Anne had done it.

Patsy and I have tried to match the example Wendy and Anne set for us since we first met them. I'm not sure we've quite reached the level the Davises achieved, but we're still trying.

Thanks Wendy. Thanks Anne. You'll probably never know what an example you gave to us. But we know. We know every day.

In early 1990, Wendy lost his beautiful bride, Anne, to cancer. Pats and I were both very sad to hear that Anne's beautiful glow had gone out. Wendy and their loving family miss her terribly, of course. The world sees only a few like Anne Davis. Thank goodness we had the chance to know her and to love her.

I talked to Wendy on the phone a few months after Anne died.

He said to me, "You know, we had a little phrase between us that we always tried to live up to, and I think we actually were able to do it. I would tell her that I loved her today, more than yesterday, but less than I would tomorrow."

"Wendy," I said, tears welling up in my eyes, "there's something that I've never told you. On the inside of our wedding rings, Pats and I had these initials inscribed, even before we were married: MTY — LTT."

On the phone there was a long pause. Then he softly said, with great warmth in his voice, "More than yesterday, less than tomorrow."

"That's right. More than yesterday, less than tomorrow. You and Anne were two very lucky people, Wendy."

"Oh, Patrick, I was the lucky one," he said. And he really meant that with his entire being.

I think they were both very lucky people to have found one another. They shared a long, good, happy life together, raised three wonderful, successful children and had a very loving and complete marriage. How much more good luck can two people possibly have in this world?

Back in Boston, in 1969, there was a hard and fast rule with all the staff of our show. When Patsy called, she was never put on hold, never asked to leave a message. No matter what I was involved with when she called, Patsy's call came before anything else or anyone else, period. Her calls were treated just like a hot line call from the White House are treated in the War Room at the Pentagon.

On the morning of our wedding anniversary I was talking to a potential guest on the phone when one of the staff told me that Patsy was on line four, calling from the hospital.

On this particular day in Boston as I reached for the phone to take Patsy's call from the hospital, I had been married to that lady for exactly ten years, almost to the hour, and yet, when I picked up the phone, I had never heard my wife sound so lost or so unable to cope.

On the other end of the line was the voice of complete desperation. This day, she would later confess, would be her lowest point in the whole saga of Michele's battle with cancer. The professionals say that there's one day in a struggle like this that you think you will not survive. June 20, 1969 was that terrible day for my Pats.

"Oh, Patrick, they want to put Michele back in the hospital today and section her lung."

I barely recognized the voice on the other end of the phone. She spoke like I might imagine her speaking if someone had been holding a loaded gun to her head.

"Why do they want to operate, Babe?"

"Doctor Tefft says that the damn spot in her lung has to be removed. He says they've tried the radiation long enough, now it's time to removed it surgically. Patrick, I just don't think I can go through any more of this. I'm at the end of the line here, Honey."

She started to cry softly into the phone.

Even now, as we look back on the whole experience, we agree that on this, the afternoon of our tenth wedding anniversary, Patsy was at the very bottom of a deep, black, bottomless hole. A hole so deep that she couldn't see any opening at the top. Her world had completely closed in on her and she was drowning. This call was not about Michele or the doctor or the operation or even that damn spot. This was not a call to inform the father of the patient what was happening. This was a frantic, desperate call for help. This was an SOS from a person who was near total collapse.

This call might just as well have been called an SYW, Save Your Wife, call instead of SOS.

As I listened to the pain and suffering and to the cry for help in Patsy's voice, I knew, in my heart, that this was one of those moments when I had to trust my instincts, above all else. It was my turn to be tough.

Something deep inside of me told me that this was also a critical moment in the whole drama of Michele. Critical for Pats, critical for me and, most of all, critical for Michele.

"Take it easy, Babe. Remember, you're not in this alone. I'm right here. Is Doctor Tefft right there with you?"

"Yes."

"Let me talk to him. Please, just hand him the phone. It's going to be alright. I promise."

"Okay."

Then I heard her say, "Patrick would like to talk to you, Doctor Tefft."

I knew I was going to have to make a very serious decision right here, right now. A decision that I couldn't discuss with my partner before I made it. Patsy was simply under too much stress at the moment to provide any clear guidance or insight for me, beyond what I had already sensed on the phone, just from the way she sounded. I was going to have to make a life and death decision for Michele, for Patsy and for our family, and I was going to have to make it alone. This day, my decision had to be the correct one. I knew it would be crucial. Somehow I also knew I wouldn't get a second chance. This was one of those times when there was no room for error.

That crafty old cancer was up to another one of its unforeseen tricks. Now, I was being asked to be a little more clever than Michele's arch enemy — the cancer that was trying to kill her.

Never forget, cancer is just that, the enemy. It's not an illness, not a disease, it's the bad guy. You must constantly remind yourself that you're dealing with a clever, deceitful, deadly enemy which must be destroyed. Your enemy must lose this game, for there is no tie in this deadly game of life and death.

I needed, here on my tenth wedding anniversary, to outsmart this foxy foe or Michele might lose the game. Which would mean that we all would lose the game. It was fourth down, goal to go, and I had just asked to be handed the ball.

"Yes," said the cool, detached, almost unfriendly voice at the other end of the line.

"Doctor Tefft?," I asked politely.

"Yes."

"Doctor Tefft, it's Patrick, Michele's dad."

"Yes."

"Give me just a moment here, if you will. I'd like to ask you a couple of questions about this spot in Michele's lung."

"Fine. What is it you'd like to know?"

His voice on the phone was flat, filled with measured patience.

Melvin Tefft knew he was not just being questioned here about a cancerous spot in a four year old child's lung. He knew he was being questioned here about his judgment as a physician. He was an eminent radiologist while I was just an uneducated civilian with only a little knowledge about medicine. It's not surprising that he was being a bit defensive.

"Has that spot shown any signs of growth in the past few weeks?"

"No, but it hasn't significantly been reduced with the radiation treatment, either, so we feel we must remove it right away, without any further delay."

"But, to answer my question, it's not growing, is it?"

"Not at this time, no," he reluctantly admitted.

"Good. Has it shown any change since the last x-rays a few weeks ago — bigger, a different shape, size, thickness? Can anything about it be seen to be new or changed, different in any way, when you compare today's film with the last ones that were taken?"

"From what we can see on the films, there doesn't seem to be any change from the last x-rays. That's why it's imperative that we remove it, surgically, at this time."

"We'll get to the operating room part of this discussion in a second. Just bear with me, if you will, Doctor. Now let me ask you this. If we watch it, x-raying Michele daily, or every other day if necessary, say, can we see if this damn spot does start to grow?"

"I would think so."

"Then can't we schedule surgery before the spot becomes a real serious threat to Michele's life?"

"Yes, I suppose that is one course of action which one might consider pursuing, Mr. Nolan. Of course it's not the option I would recommend at this stage in Michele's treatment, however."

"I fully understand your position, Doctor. Thank you for your candor. Now, Doctor Tefft, I want you to do me a great big favor. I want you to please take a very close look at your whole patient, which includes the lady you have there before you. Take a very, very close look at her, Doctor, please. The lady before you is being asked to do more than anyone should be asked to do. She's been hauling Michele back and forth to Boston every day for months, worried sick that she might lose her baby daughter. She's been taking care of her family every day and now, at thirty-four years of age, she's about to give birth to her third child, as you can plainly see. In fact, today, Doctor Tefft, is not only our wedding anniversary, but it's the actual due date for the baby she's carrying. That's an exhausted lady you have standing there before you, Doctor Tefft.

"Now, without thinking about any of that," I continued, not waiting for a reply, "you tell her that you've decided that the best course of action is to put her four year old baby in the hospital and have Bob Filler chop a chunk out of one of her lungs.

"Doctor, you're quite simply not looking at the whole picture here. Good as she is, that lady before you simply can't be in two places at once.

"You've looked at an x-ray plate and made a medical decision. You've decided that surgery is unquestionably indicated, at this time, at this stage, in this case. Look a little more closely, if you will, Doctor, at your whole patient. Look very carefully, Doctor. Part of your patient is thirty-four years old, very weary and very, very pregnant. We've got to make a human decision here about people, not just a medical call based on percentages and probabilities."

Silence on the phone. He wasn't backing down for a minute. A disrespectful civilian was telling him how to practice medicine. He didn't like that one little bit, so he just remained silent. A lot of them do that when you disagree with their judgment. They just stand silently, waiting for you to blink. I was in no mood to blink this day.

"Now, Doctor Tefft. ... are you still there?"

"Yes."

"Swell. Here's what we're going to do today, Doctor. Here's our course of action.

"You're going to tell that very pregnant lady to bundle up her four year old baby and take her home. We're going to check on that spot in a couple of days. If it's growing, we'll talk about operating. If it isn't, we'll look at it again in another couple of days, but today we're not going to schedule surgery. Today, Doctor Tefft, Michele and her mother are going to go home."

"Mr. Nolan, you understand then that this is your decision and that Michele is then your responsibility?"

He said this veiled threat in a cold, clinical manner. A manner which really annoyed me.

He was trying to intimidate me with guilt by telling me that I would be to blame for whatever happened as a result of my decision not to let him have his way and operate on Michele.

"Now you listen to me and you listen very, very carefully, Doctor Tefft," I said as strongly and forcefully as I could — without raising my voice.

"Michele has always been our responsibility. We've never asked you, or anyone else at the Jimmy Fund, to take on that responsibility. We've only asked that you provide the best possible medical care and your best advice. The responsibility has always been with us, her parents. I wish to hell that you medical people would one day get that straight, just once."

"Just as long as we understand each other," he said, still not listening to me.

"We understand each other perfectly, Doctor. You want to do what's clinically next in line and I want to see that the whole patient is given the most reasonable and responsible care. Now, send my wife and her babies home. I've got work to do and you and I don't have anything more to talk to each other about today.

"But before you do that, Doctor, I want to make one other thing perfectly clear to you. I want you to make no editorial comments about this conversation to my wife after we hang up. She's carrying all the load she can carry right now. If you add one more item, one more than you

119

already have, to that load, I'll come down to the clinic and we'll have another a little chat, but this time it will be face to face. And let me assure you, Doctor, you do not want to have that conversation with me. Not today you don't. You can think, to yourself, that I'm a roaring asshole, but you'd better not share that opinion with Patsy. Not today."

Patsy came back on the line and through her tears she thanked me and wished me a happy anniversary, again.

"Now take your two babies and go home. Are you sure you're all right to drive? If you're not, I'll come right over to Childrens and drive you home myself," I said.

"We'll be fine, honey. I'm okay, honest. Michele and I will see you at home tonight," she said. "I love you, very much."

"I'll be about and hour and a half behind you. I'm almost wrapped up here. Drive carefully. I love you, too. Tell Michele that her dad loves her."

"We both love you," she barely whispered into the phone through her tears.

Her voice seemed a little less stressed out than when she first called, but only just a little less desperate. It was only just a barely perceivable improvement. She was very relieved that Michele was going home today and not to surgery, but she still didn't have a great deal of rope left.

Personally, I was furious at that guy Melvin Tefft for putting her in that position. Here, it seemed, we had another brilliant medical clinician who seemed to possess the bedside manner of a blind frog.

Never, not even for one second, did I second guess myself on the decision I made that day about Michele's surgery. I knew it was the right thing to do. I knew it was the only thing we could do. I knew it then, I knew it six weeks later and I know it now, as I write about it some twenty years later. Sometimes you have to trust your instincts completely, without any second guessing. This was one of those times.

As Thomas Jefferson once so eloquently said, "Make sure you're right, then go ahead."

That same night, as a somewhat somber tenth anniversary dinner was coming to a close, Bob Filler called. Before he could say a word, I jumped all over him. I told him that if he was calling to tell me to bring Michele to the hospital in the morning so he could cut a piece out of her lung, he was going to be very disappointed.

"I'm not bringing Michele in tomorrow, Bob. Period. I'm very serious."

"I know you are. But will you please relax and listen for a minute, Patrick?"

"Sorry."

"Just calm down for a second," he went on. "I'm calling to tell you that you're absolutely right about Michele and that damn spot. The last thing I'd do, at this stage of her treatment, is to operate on her lung. Of course we're going to watch it. Of course we can take it out later, if we need to do that at all. I just wanted you to know that I'm completely on your side. You're right. Doctor Tefft is wrong, this time."

I relaxed a bit. "Have you spoken to Tefft?"

"Oh, yes, and I've told him what I've just told you. It's simple, this time, he's wrong. As you, apparently very eloquently, told him this morning, we can watch that spot for weeks. If it starts to change or grow, we'll talk about surgery. Right now, Michele's right where she belongs — at home.

"How's she doing?" he asked.

"She's asleep. She ate fairly well tonight, but she's getting tired of the whole thing, but not as tired as Patsy is," I said.

"How is the mother-to-be doing?"

"She's feeling better, thanks. I fixed her a nice dinner. She'll be very happy to know you called, thanks.

"Now, if we can just get the new baby to wake up and get moving. Pats is really sick of being pregnant, Bob. It's been a long nine months. Today's her due date, in fact," I told him.

"Yes, it has been a long, tiring pregnancy for her. But, neither you nor I can really understand or appreciate what going through all this has been like for her. I know I'm not strong enough to have done what she's been doing," Bob said, flatly.

I agreed with him. I wasn't either.

"I'm fairly sure I'm not strong enough to even be pregnant, much less be pregnant while a child of mine is being treated for cancer," Bob said.

"Neither am I, Bob. She's really a wonder. Thanks for your support. I really appreciate it, a lot. Probably much more than you'll never know," I told him.

"Let us know when the baby's born. I understand the two of you are doing it at home? You're both okay about that are you?"

"Just fine. In fact, that's the least of the worries around here. I'll let you know. It should be any time now, I hope."

"Maybe you should have been a doctor instead of a television producer," he joked.

"Are you kidding? Most of you doctors think I'm such a royal pain in the butt that I never would have lived through the first year of medical school. I'd have been found hanging by my ears down in the morgue one morning with a tag on my toe."

Bob was laughing on the other end of the line.

"But, thanks for the compliment, Bob. See ya later, and thanks, again, for the call," I said.

"You're more than welcome. Please give Patsy my best. Tell her to get some rest."

"I will. Thanks for calling, Bob. Good night."

He rang off. After he did, I sat there for a few minutes thinking how I was, once again, so pleased that we had a doctor on our side who wasn't afraid to contradict the opinion of one of his colleagues and agree with the parents. Bob Filler is a wonderful physician and a good friend. He would continue to prove that in the weeks and months which were still ahead for us.

Patrick came in and told me that Bob Filler had just called and agreed with us that surgery on Michele's lung was not indicated. I was greatly relieved. I knew we were doing the right thing, for all of us, but it sure was wonderful to hear that we weren't alone in that conviction.

That night, I slept a lot better than I had in a while, but I was so large with child that I had to sit up just to turn over. Patrick had long ago

121

moved out of our bed and onto the couch. He just couldn't sleep with the awkward water buffalo anymore. God, how I wanted this kid to be born.

Two days later (the day that would have been Michele's first day, post surgery, had we consented to the lung surgery), I felt what I thought might be the first advance notices from my uterus that it was getting as tired as I was of the load we were both carrying. It turned out to be a night of false labor, but the following afternoon, when the contractions returned, I knew that at last, this was the real thing.

By three in the afternoon I knew that before long we would have three children in our family. I also hoped we would be able to hang onto number two.

Our first child had been born in Hawaii, the second one in California and this, the last one, would be born at 6 Old Meadow Road, Sudbury, Massachusetts 01776.

It had been mutually decided by Patrick and me, months ago, that this third child would be our last child. As it turned out, he was the last one we produced, but he wasn't the last child to join our family.

A few weeks before the baby was due, the executive producer at WBZ, Mel Bernstein, called Patrick in and asked if the station could film the birth, with plans to broadcast it as a "special," prime time, program.

Patrick was thrilled, but he told Mel that the decision was much more my decision than his. Mel told him that whatever I decided was fine, but that the station thought our home birth, with the father delivering the baby, would be a very powerful and dramatic story. Patrick, of course, agreed.

After some discussion, I decided that it would be all right for a small crew to come to the house and film the birth. But I had just two ironclad conditions.

The first condition was that they simply record what happened. They were not to try to direct or control what we did, nor were they, in any way, to involve themselves in the birth of the baby or in any of the birthing activities. If there wasn't enough light or if someone wasn't sitting in the right place — tough. They were to be silent, unobtrusive observers of the event — like flies on the wall.

Second, and to me, most important, if for any reason — or for no reason — I suddenly wanted them out of the room, they would leave without discussion. All I had to do was say, "GO," and they would be gone.

WBZ and Mel agreed to all my conditions, as did the two cameramen, Jim Arnold and John Premack who had volunteered to record our baby's arrival, when we met with them a few days later.

So, when I was sure that we were actually on the baby track, I had Patrick call John and Jim, who were waiting for our call.

Earlier I had told them not to drop what they were doing and rush to the house when Patrick called. This wasn't one of those fires which they so enjoyed filming. Labor and delivery had taken several hours on the other two occasions when I had babies, this one wasn't going to be over in a flash. I knew from the past that we were all in for a long, sleepless night.

John and Jim arrived at our house about nine that evening with their cameras and lights.

Patsy's labor, as it had been with Michele's, four years earlier, took all night. This time, however, there wasn't any battle with hospital administrators, nurses or controlling doctors. This night was our night.

As the night turned into morning, it was evident that we were bogged down, again, as we had been with Michele's birth. Patsy had moved what she thought was the baby down the birth canal and struggled to ease that load into the daylight.

For the last three hours I had been sitting on the bed, between Patsy's legs, looking for signs of a baby to appear. At last I saw something.

"Pats, I don't think what I'm seeing is the baby's head."

"It has to be. I'm working as hard as I can and it feels like it's about to be born."

I didn't want to tell her what I saw, but I knew, without a whole lot of doubt, that I was seeing not the baby's bald head, but the thick layers of film that composed the baby's amniotic sac. It wasn't a baby. We were having a bag of cloudy water.

"Pats. It's the amniotic sac down in the birth canal. I just saw a swirl of fluid during that contraction."

"Oh, Jesus."

She knew she had moved not the baby, but a bag of water through transition. Her work was far from done.

"I think if I take this clamp and tear a hole in it, like that doctor did when we were having Michele, that we'll be okay."

She sat up on her elbows and looked right into my face. "Are you sure it's the sac?"

"Yes. I'm sure, honey."

"Then go ahead," she said, laying back against the pillows and the cushions that I had put behind her back on the bed.

I picked up the clean pair of forceps we had standing by to clamp the cord with and pressed them against the straining membranes of the sac that held our baby prisoner. Moment of truth, I thought, as I pinched it.

"Eureka!," I shouted, as an explosion of amniotic fluid and a water drenched the front of me. "We struck oil, Babe."

The pressure had been enormous. I was wet from my chin to my knees. I was elated, but Patsy was almost despondent.

"I can't do this. I just can't do this anymore," she said, falling back.

A flash of panic ran through my soul. If she was finished, what the hell were we going to do. This baby was yet to be born. I knew that my only hope of bringing Patsy back into focus was to get her angry at me.

"What the hell do mean you can't do this? Who the hell do you think is going to do it. You can't quit now."

"I have to. I'm beat. I just can't do it any more."

"Bullshit. You started this thing, lady, and now you're going to finish it. You're not the only one who's been working here all night, you know. I'm bushed, too. I want to quit, but I can't quit and neither can you, damn it. What do you want me to tell everybody? That you're a quitter?"

She sat up on her elbows again and glared at me.

"You've been working hard? You're tired? You're ready to quit? Let me tell you something ..."

She never finished that sentence. The next contraction, now that the pressure in her womb was relieved, slammed her back into the pillows and cushions. All she could utter was a deep, low growl. The baby had ended the argument, his own way.

"I knew you weren't a quitter," I said softly.

Actually she didn't have any choice. The baby, now without a big bubble of water in his way, was headed for daylight at near light speed. Things now, as they had with Michele's birth after the release of fluids, would move right along.

Since the baby had remained in the amniotic fluid through the long hours of labor, he had not had an opportunity to dry out. With all of nature's lubrication still covering his body and the powerful new contractions from Mom, that baby should slide right down the birth canal. And he did. Before we knew it, his head crowned.

"He's here, babe. This time it's not sac, it's baby. A baby's big, hairy head. Take it easy now, just relax and wait for the next contraction. You're doing great. Take it easy. We're about to become parents again."

I continued to encourage her and coax her into relaxing as I watched this unbelievable event unfold right in front of me, between our legs.

Sure enough, with the next contraction, which wasn't as strong, the baby's head fell into my waiting hand. Patsy laid back on her pillows and gasped for breath.

"Easy, babe. Easy does it. Just relax now. The head's out. We're almost there."

"Is he out?," she asked, knowing he wasn't, but hoping she was wrong.

"Just his head. Next contraction. He's rolling on his side, just like the book said he would."

Without any help from me, that baby performed the most perfect ninety degree roll to the left so that his shoulders could more easily fit through the snug opening and over Patsy's pelvic bones.

Thinking back to Michele's birth, I remembered how bluish she had looked before she had taken her first breath of fresh air.

The baby's head that I was now holding in the palm of my hand was clearly blue. Pale, reddish blue. He didn't look alive, but I knew he was. It was very strange to be holding a motionless, blue baby's head in your hand for the first time.

"Take it easy. Take it easy, babe. Don't bear down. Just relax, it's going to happen as soon as we get another contraction. I think you're just about finished with your night's work, honey. Here we go."

I didn't need to tell her. She knew better than anyone else in the room that her uterus was about to expel its precious cargo, at long last.

As the next, very gentle contraction started, so did the baby's progress. As easily as a wet bar of soap would slip from a lathered hand, the baby slid out of his mother and into the waiting hands of his father. He was, as he should have been, face down, his back to me.

As I held him up by his very slippery ankles, Patsy's first words were, "My God, he's an elephant, but he's a boy."

"You're kidding?," I said as I spun him around so I could confirm his external plumbing equipment.

"He sure is. Hello, Patrick Henry Nolan, the seventh. Welcome to the world," I almost shouted.

What a feeling that was. I'll never, ever forget that moment as long as I live.

As I eased this new little Patrick down onto his mother's stomach so we could clear his mouth and nose of the fluid and mucus, he performed his first act as a new, little human being. He peed on his father.

"Thanks, a lot, kid," I said through the tears of joy that were freely rolling down my cheeks.

Then I watched as the most amazing thing happened. At first, there was a blue baby, laying quite still on his mother's stomach. But as I began to wipe away the fluid from his face and suction out his nose and mouth with a small rubber syringe, he started to fill his lungs on his own. The oxygen flowed into his lungs and enriched his blood, for the first time with his own breath, and he turned from blue to pink then to rosy, healthy bright red and then slowly back to bright, healthy pink.

He was just fine. He had all his toes and fingers. He was outside and he was breathing and he was alive and I was the father of a beautiful son. Somewhere the birds were singing. Somewhere a band was playing. There was joy in Mudville.

When we were sure that he was breathing fine, I eased him up to his mother's breast. The human body, being the marvelous machine that it is, needed a clue that the baby was outside the womb before it released the placenta from the inside of his mother's womb. With his first attempt to suckle, another powerful contraction of the uterus expelled a huge placenta and it's now useless amniotic sac and cord. What a mess we now had in the middle of our bed.

Suddenly I remembered. I had the job of cleaning this all up.

"Now what?," I asked, suddenly becoming the giddy, slap happy, excited new father, nearly unable to think clearly.

"Just relax," said the now in charge, completely relaxed obstetrical nurse. "We're not done just yet."

I took the clamp, and with a little direction from my assistant, stripped the blood with my hand back down the cord into Patrick — just as I remembered seeing the doctor in Bakersfield do with Michele — and then I clamped off the bluish, now unneeded umbilical cord a few inches from Patrick.

Picking up the soft, woven umbilical tape Patsy had brought home from the hospital I asked, "Which side do I tie this on?"

"On the him side," she calmly said.

"Right. The him side. About here?"

"That should do just fine. No granny knots now."

"Right! No grannies," I said.

Suddenly I realized that the new mother was calmly making jokes.

"Easy for you to say," I said. "You're not trying to tie a knot with this greasy stuff all over your hands."

I could barely hold onto the tape it was so slippery from the lubrication that had covered Patrick.

"Is that baby here yet?," came the query from the doorway.

Michele was tired of waiting and had come to see if a baby had been born.

"He just arrived, sweetie. Say hello to Patrick, your new little brother."

125

"A brother? I told you I wanted another sister."

"Sorry, they had a special on brothers today and that's what you got."

"Is the baby here?" came another voice from the hallway.

It was Teresa with a couple of her friends. Apparently, I thought, word spreads fast out there on Old Meadow Lane.

"Yes. Patrick is right here," Pats told her.

"Dad, I want to see that cord," Teresa said.

A few weeks before he was born, Teresa had asked me one of the most interesting questions any seven year old had ever asked about the birthing process.

I had been shaving at about six o'clock one morning, before heading out to work. Teresa came into the bathroom, still a little groggy with sleep.

"I've been wondering about this baby we're going to have," she had said.

"Yes," I said. "What can I do for you, Charlie?"

Like a cat, she climbed up on the counter beside the sink and sat looking up at me as I continued to shave.

"Well," she said, "I think I understand how he got in there and I think I understand how he's going to get out, but will you please tell me something that's really been bothering me?"

"Sure," I said, feeling a little curious about what could be so important to have gotten her up at this hour to ask me about.

"Well," she said, "you told me how he eats while he's in there and I know he sleeps in there, but will you please tell me how he goes to the bathroom while he's in there?"

"Piece of cake. Do you know where the baby book is?"

She hopped down from the counter and went to get the book on babies that we had used for the girls prenatal instruction about their new sibling.

When she returned, she climbed up and stood on the toilet so we could look at the book together. I had her open the book to the page which dealt with the ninth month of gestation. There was a color drawing of a fully formed embryo in the womb, at full term.

"See the cord?"

"Yeah. That's how he eats and how he gets air," she said, with all the confidence of an old hand at baby making.

"That's right. That's also how he goes to the bathroom before he's born. Just like Mom has to eat his food and breath his air and then pass them down the cord into the baby, the cord returns to Mom all the waste products from the baby. You know how often she's been running to the bathroom lately?"

"Every ten minutes. Dad, we had to stop on the way to the hospital last week — twice" Teresa said a bit impatiently.

"Try sleeping with her," I offered.

"See, if you look real close, you can see that the cord is actually two cords, twisted together. One is for food and oxygen going in, the other is for waste and water and bad air coming out."

"So Mom has to go to the bathroom for him, too?"

"In a sense, yes," I said.

"Did she have to do that for me and Michele, too?"

"That's the way it works, kid."

"Well, when this baby's born, I'd like to see that cord."

"Fine by me. Anything else bothering you?"

She looked up at me as I resumed shaving and said, "I don't think so. I sure wish this baby would hurry up and get here though."

"I know just how you feel, I can hardly wait myself. But Mom's the one who really needs to have that baby get here."

Teresa looked up at me as she slowly closed the book, satisfied for the moment that she was on top of the action. Then she said, "She sure does get cranky sometimes lately."

"She needs all the help we can give her around here and all the support we can muster. This making babies business is tough stuff, kid. It makes you very tired. Just wait. One day you'll see for yourself.

(As we were writing this book, Teresa and her husband, Ted produced a beautiful baby girl. They named the baby Lillian, after Patsy's Mom. We were very pleased.)

"We need to do all we can to give Mom a hand around here. And when the baby arrives there'll be even more for you to do."

"Dad. Is this baby a boy or a girl?"

"Yes!" I said firmly, kissing her on the head as I walked out of the bathroom, turning off the lights as I went.

"Hey, wait for me."

Now that day had finally arrived. The baby was here, it was a boy and Teresa wanted to make sure that her father had told her the truth about how the baby had gone to the bathroom in the womb.

First, I showed her the big part of the cord which was still attached to the placenta, then the part that was still attached to Patrick, still being held in his mother's arms.

"It sure is a funny looking thing, all blue and strange," she said, looking at the stub of a cord that protruded from Patrick's round, pink tummy.

"Exactly what I thought, when I first saw Michele's," I said.

"What happens now? Do we have to cut off the rest of it in a few days?"

I smiled, "Nope. In a couple of days, probably a week or so, it will just fall off and he'll have a regular belly button, just like yours."

"He is kind of cute, Dad."

"I thought you'd like him."

I looked around the room. There were at least ten kids milling around, including Pam Adams in a full football uniform with shoulder pads and helmet, looking at the baby and giggling.

"Would you get all these kids out of here, please. I'd like to take a shower," Patsy said.

"You feel up to a shower? You've only been a mother for about fifteen minutes. Don't you want to take a few minutes and catch your breath?"

"I'm greasy and sticky and sweaty and yucky and I want to take a shower and go to sleep for three days. I'd like you to help me into the bathroom and then change the bed," she said, as she started to sit up, carefully moving baby Patrick onto the bed beside her.

"Sure. Hang on. Let me get rid of all your fans, first. Okay, gang. It's time to hit the road. I'll let you see Patrick a little later today. Right now the new mommy has to get some rest and so does the baby."

They all obediently trooped out of our bedroom and went back outside to resumed playing. It was just another quiet summer's day for the gang on Old Meadow Road in Sudbury, Massachusetts.

So there it was, finally all done. At around ten o'clock on the morning of June twenty-fifth, nineteen hundred and sixty nine, we had all been thrilled to welcome into the world, Patrick Henry Nolan, VII, who weighed in at around eight, rosy red pounds. A healthy, happy baby boy. Wow.

That day was one of the greatest days of my life. The day I delivered my own son. But, my heavens, what a mess. As I'd agreed, I did clean it all up. Patsy got up a few minutes after the baby was born and took a shower. When she returned, John and Jim and I had made the bed with clean, dry sheets. She smiled at us, looked around the room and told us all, gently, but firmly, to leave.

"And, please, take that baby with you. I'm going to get some sleep now," she told us.

Jim and John, who had only met Patsy briefly at a couple of social functions associated with the Ad Club or the station and then at our pre-birth production meeting, were not at all close to her before this night. But, as they were about to leave, both of them came over to the bed and lovingly kissed her goodbye. Here were two hardcore, "I've seen it all" television news cameramen with tears in their eyes as they congratulated Patsy, telling her how proud they both were to share this special moment with her. They were both as impressed with my lady, and what she had done this day, as I was. Jim Arnold, particularly, remains very fond of Patsy to this day.

The last time I saw him, sixteen years after our "blessed event," the first thing he asked me was, "How's my friend, Patsy?" He wanted me to be sure to remember him to her when I got home. I was pleased to do that for him. She was pleased that he remembered her. Remember her? How could he ever forget her?

Westinghouse eventually had some reservations about broadcasting a program which might promote unassisted childbirth at home, so the program never aired. I did use a piece of the film on my morning show the day after Patrick was born, so both my oldest and my youngest children were on television within twenty-four hours of having been born. Teresa, in Hawaii on the evening news, and Patrick, in Boston on New England Today. (I had been working for a radio station when Michele was born so I could only tell everyone in the San Joaquin Valley that she had joined the world. Later, she would have her day on TV.)

As the guys were saying goodbye to Pats, I took Patrick and went out to the living room to call the Grandparents from cloud nine. Zowie, what a day it had been — and it wasn't even noon yet.

Within days, Little Patrick joined the team which traveled to Boston each day. He quickly become the favorite of everyone at the Jimmy Fund. Patrick was always such a happy baby. He's a happy young man to this day, always seeing the bright side, always with an amusing one-liner about something. He's still a joy to his father's heart, as he was that morning in our bedroom in Sudbury.

Little did we know when he was born, however, that Patrick's mere presence would quickly become a major problem for us.

But then, after that last spot in her lung vanished from the x-ray plates a few weeks after Patrick was born, we didn't think that we were ever going to have to contend with Michele's cancer again, either.

The doctors had decided to use a stronger, more directed beam of radiation on that damn spot, rather than operate and remove it surgically. Within a few days, the x-ray films showed that all traces of that stubborn spot of cancer in her left lung had vanished.

Old "Slick," however, still had one more surprise up his sleeve. We'd been pretty clever, up to now, but we'd need a real good magician to make our enemy's last, fiendish trick, fail.

If we thought kidney cancer in a three year old and cancerous spots in her lungs and exploratory surgery on a four year old were serious, we were in for a big surprise. The worst — and the best — were both yet to come.

And come they would, within weeks of Patrick's marvelous birth at home.

*I turned toward Patsy and was about to start quizzing her
on what had happened here this morning
when I heard Jaffe say to the clerk,
"Please call Doctor Filler and ask him
to come over right away.
He seems to be the only one here
who can handle Mister Nolan."*

Chapter Eight

"It's Only A Small Headache, Mom!"

After I delivered our son Patrick at home, I started daily brainwashing sessions with our pal, Charlie Austin.

Charlie and his sweet wife, Linda, were just about to welcome their second child into the world and I wanted him to be there for the big event. With, Lisa, their first baby, Charlie had wanted no part of what he called, "Woman's work" — the birthing process. He didn't mind, as he said, being there for the laying of the keel, but when it came time to the launch, that was "woman's work."

When I showed him some of the film of Patrick's birth and after he was bombarded by my daily lectures on where a Father belongs when his child is born, he agreed to have a talk with Linda's obstetrician about sharing the experience.

When Patrick was four weeks old, I got a call from Charlie one afternoon.

"Man, you were right on. It was the greatest experience of my life. Linda and I have never been closer after going through this together. I owe you, Man. I really owe you," just flowed out of the phone.

"Charlie, is it a girl or a boy?," I asked calmly.

"The most beautiful little girl you have ever seen in your life, Man. She's just gorgeous," he said with great, fatherly pride.

"Linda's doing well?"

"Linda is a champion. Listen. That lady is the strongest, smartest, toughest, meanest, best woman in the world. My God, how I love that lady," said Charlie, the guy who four weeks ago didn't want to be anywhere near where a baby was being born.

"Congratulation. Give your lady a kiss for us. Now, wasn't I right? No one can tell you how great an experience it is until you do it. You have to be there yourself, don't you?"

"Absolutely! I never, never in my wildest dreams, could have imagined feeling this way. It was the best. Thanks. I owe you," he said in his deep, baritone voice.

"I'll collect," I said with a grin, not knowing how soon I would actually be repaid for my lectures and brainwashings and scoldings.

On Friday, the fifteenth of August, Michele, the new baby Patrick and I were at the Jimmy Fund for one of Michele's regular checkups. The x-rays were clear, except for that small, stubborn shadow in her lung, the blood tests were normal and everything looked great when she went in to be examined by Dr. Traggis.

"How are you feeling, Michele?," he asked.

"Fine, thank you," she answered, holding a small piece of cotton on the finger where they had just drawn the blood sample.

"She's complained of a headache this morning," I told him.

"It's just a little headache, Mom," Michele said, casually.

"Does it hurt right now?," asked the Doctor.

"No."

"When does it hurt?"

"Just once in a while."

"Does it hurt for a long time?"

"No, it's just a little headache," she calmly assured him.

He took out an ophthalmoscope and asked her to look straight at his forehead. Michele was always amazing with those eye examinations. She would hold very still and look directly ahead. They were always able to get a real good look at her retina.

Doctor Traggis looked at both of her eyes, carefully, just as he did everything, before he said,"I don't see any pressure at all. I would keep a close eye on her over the weekend and if there's any change, or if the headaches get worse in any way, please call me on Monday."

"What could be causing these brief, little headaches?," I asked

"Could be a reaction to the medicine. Could be a sinus pressure thing. It could be a lot of things, but without anything else to go on, we'll just have to watch her closely."

"I just get a little scared whenever something different happens," I said to this man I had grown to know and care so much about.

He looked up at me and as our eyes met he said, "I know. I'm just like you. We've done so well for the last few weeks that anything new scares me to death."

"Can we go home how, Mom?," asked Michele.

"Yes, dear. Let's get your brother and head for home."

We drove back out Route Nine to 128 and then north to The Boston Post Road — Route 20, toward Sudbury. It was a lovely, late summer's day, cool and crisp, bright and clear.

On that trip home she said twice that her head hurt, but each time only lasted for a few seconds before she was fine. It was as if a switch would be thrown and the pain would suddenly appear. Seconds later, it would just as suddenly disappear. It was very strange. I was only slightly concerned. Maybe it was just the change in pressure as the climate started to move New England toward fall. I hoped that's all it was.

On Saturday morning she was walking across the living room floor and suddenly laid down flat as a pancake and didn't move.

"Are you all right?," Patrick asked.

She didn't answer, but just lay there with her eyes open, not moving. In a few seconds she got up and continued across the floor.

"Are you okay?," he asked, again.

"Yes. I just had a little headache, Daddy," she told him very matter of factually.

"It's gone?"

"Yes. I'm fine now, Daddy," she said as she went on toward her room.

I had told Patrick about the headaches when he got home the night before. As usual, he was scared something was wrong, again. Even though Michele seemed to have slept fine throughout the night, I thought the headaches were a little longer in induration this morning. And, maybe, a little more frequent.

"Is she okay, Pats?" he asked me with more than a little concern in his voice.

"I don't know, honey. They couldn't see any pressure in her eyes. She doesn't have a temperature or any other symptoms. I don't know what to make of these little headaches. She just lays down and doesn't move for a few seconds and then she's fine again. It's very strange," I said, holding back the dread I felt building in the pit of my stomach.

The little headaches didn't seem to inhibit her play or other activities, she'd just lay down and stay very still when she felt one of them coming on. They were almost like a wave of pain and would quickly build, break over her and then be gone. We didn't know what to make of it. Michele, of course, like everything else in her life, took these little headaches in stride, never fussing about them or seeming even to be concerned about them.

Saturday night the headaches seemed to have gotten longer in duration and, although we didn't time them, they seemed to be more frequent, too. I got up several times during the night to check on her. She slept through the night, but her sleep was somewhat restless.

On Sunday morning the headaches went from being little headaches to being serious headaches. I called the Jimmy Fund.

After a ten minute chat with the doctor I found on call, we decided that bringing her in to the hospital wasn't the wisest thing to do. They'd just admit her to Childrens and then watch her until Monday morning when the Jimmy Fund doctors could examine her. We could watch her much better and much more closely here at home. There were no technicians or lab people at the Jimmy Fund on Sunday to do any of the tests, so we agreed that waiting until the first thing Monday morning was the best course of action.

Sunday night we got almost no sleep as one or the other of us was up checking on Michele every half hour or so. She seemed to sleep, but it was a fitful, uncomfortable sleep. Several times she cried out in her sleep.

Dawn found me sitting in Grandma's old rocking chair, holding her and gently rocking her.

"What's the plan, Babe?," Patrick asked at five-thirty.

"I'll take her in and be at the Jimmy Fund at eight when the doctors arrive," I said.

"What about Patrick?"

"He can go with me. He's fine, just as long as his personal cow is not too far away."

133

Patrick smiled.

The baby Patrick was six weeks old and was not at all interested in anything that came from a bottle. If it wasn't milk from my breast, he rejected it. With the first two children I had been able to breast feed them for only a few weeks before demand overcame production. This time, however — maybe I was more relaxed about it — I seemed to be producing all he needed. And this kid needed a lot.

"I'll go in, do the show and see you at the Jimmy Fund as soon as I can. If there's anything to tell me before I get there, call me at the station. You have the direct line to the booth and the news room number just in case that phone's busy, right?," he asked.

"I have the numbers. Besides, Gladys would leave the board and track you down in the bathroom if I asked her to."

Patrick nodded through a smile.

Gladys was a wonderful woman of about sixty who had operated the WBZ switchboard for over twenty years. She had taken a liking to Patrick and when I took the baby in to visit him, she fell in love with yet another Patrick.

I called the station a lot that summer, so Gladys and I became well acquainted. She could find Patrick when no one else had a clue as to where he was. Once she rang the scenic shop and found him there discussing a special set with the carpenter. His office had said he was out of the building, but Gladys couldn't remember seeing him pass her little window on the way to the parking lot. If he had left the building, Gladys would have seen him.

"OK. Are you sure you want to deal with the baby? Maybe I should take him to the studio with me," he offered.

"Honey, you're good at a lot of things, but you can't feed him."

"Okay. Call me as soon as you talk to the doctors," he said heading out to the car and to the forty minute drive to WBZ.

"I will. I promise," I promised as he closed the door.

To say that my mind was not on the Broadway star, the live news maker report from Dorchester, the weather report, the movie review and the other elements that made up the New England Today show that day, would be a gross understatement. Fortunately I had a great group of people working with me and, that morning, they carried the ball.

Our co-hosts were Joe Harper and Pat Collins. (not the nightclub hypnotist, the TV film critic you see quoted in movie ads all the time.) They were two great people with whom to work.

That morning, the direct line in the booth rang before we were off the air. It was Patsy telling me that they had done some blood tests and found nothing abnormal. They had looked in her eyes and they were surprised that she was still able to see with all the pressure she had developed behind her eyes. They didn't know how she could still be conscious. Michele, we both knew, was in trouble, again.

"There seems to be a great deal of swelling in her head. They don't know why. We're going to have some x-rays, they're going to do a EEG and then they want to do what's called a brain scan, about noon," she said.

"Do you want me to come right over?"

"When you're done. What I do need you to do is take care of Patrick while I go to x-ray with Michele."

"Are they going to admit Michele to the hospital?"

"They already have. Bob Filler took care of it," she said.

"Is he worried?," I wanted to know

"He's concerned and confused."

"Confused? About what?," I wanted to know.

"He says that Wilm's never moves to the brain. There's something called the blood brain barrier. They don't really understand how it works, but some drugs and some diseases just never pass through that barrier to affect the brain. Wilm's, historically, is one of those types of cancer that never moves to the brain.

"So he's confused and so are all the rest of the people here at the Jimmy Fund. That's why we're going to do the x-rays and that's why they've scheduled a brain scan," she told me.

"What the hell is a brain scan and what's an EEG?," I wanted to know.

"An EEG is an Electroencephalogram and a brain scan, as I understand it, is a heat sensitive picture of the brain — a new type of special x-ray, I guess," she offered.

"Where will I find you when I get there?," I wanted to be sure I didn't have to run around in that huge complex trying to find them in x-ray, the lab, the hospital or wherever.

"When will you be here?"

"I'll be there at ten-fifteen, sooner if you want," I told her.

"There's no rush. I'll meet you here at the Jimmy Fund with Patrick. He can't go anywhere over at Childrens except the lobby," she reminded me.

In those days a small child only went upstairs if they were admitted as a patient. Things have changed a little, but there were strict rules about children visitors, back in 1969.

"Do you want me to come right now"

"No. We're just waiting for the doctor to check her eyes, again. I'll see you at ten-fifteen. Don't park, just pull in out front. You're going to take Patrick back to your office for a while, aren't you?"

"If you don't need me there with you."

"Michele and I'll be fine. I can call you when we know something. There's not much to do here really but wait," she said, completely relaxed and in control.

She was worried, but she was in complete charge of her emotions. This time, unlike the scare with the lung surgery, Pats was well rested, no longer pregnant and able to be strong, no matter what was ahead of us. It's that amazing inner strength that got us through the tough spots. We'd need it again, before this day was over.

"Be sure you've stuffed that little bugger as full as you can before I get there. I'll see you in twenty minutes or so. I love you."

"I love you, too. I'm going to feed him right now. Drive carefully," she said as she hung up.

I finished the show, which seemed to take another three hours, and told the staff that we would have our production meeting on tomorrow's show when I got back. I tried to dash past Gladys, but she stopped me.

"Is everything OK? You look a little frazzled, Patrick," she observed.

"Michele's having some headaches and we're trying to find out what they're all about. That's all. I'm going over to Childrens right now. But I do have some good news for you. I'm bringing the baby back for a while."

Her face lit up, "Wonderful. He's such a happy little thing."

I left and drove over to Jamaica Plain where the Jimmy Fund was located. Traffic was light and I made it fairly quickly. Of course, any drive in the City of Boston is an adventure, no matter what time of day it might be.

I picked up Patrick, gave Pats a quick kiss and headed back to BZ. I had lots of work to do on the show. Producing a live magazine or talk show every day is a little close to complete madness. Only those who's personalities border on the insane should ever get involved in one. It can make you old in a hurry.

There were the guests who didn't show, or who couldn't talk much past, yep and nope, or the ones I used to love the most. The authors or other non performers who sounded so articulate and lucid on the phone when you booked them who, when they got on the air, clammed up and couldn't express a coherent reply to the question, "How are you." It made for long minutes of live television.

But, today, we had guests to book, ideas to discuss, a production meeting to chair and a near famous little six week old baby boy for everyone in the building to fuss over. It was a totally unproductive two hours.

Before noon, Patrick was screaming his head off for his personal milk supply. It was time to head back to Childrens and get him some warm lunch.

I parked the car in the small lot near the clinic and took the back stairs up through the old side building of the Jimmy Fund. I crossed over the bridge on the second floor and came out in Childrens Hospital just down the hall from the x-ray department where I had agreed to meet Patsy during the noon hour. She was nowhere to be seen.

"Do you know where Patsy Nolan is?," I asked an x-ray technician.

"Yes. She and her daughter are in number three," she indicted a room down the side hall that began the labyrinth of passageways, x-ray rooms, dark rooms, viewing rooms and waiting rooms in the x-ray department.

"Thank you."

"He sounds hungry," she said, referring to my small companion's bright red face and healthy lungs.

By now, Patrick was really screaming his head off.

"I'm trying to fix that," I said, ducking down the passageway toward the room with a big three on the door.

Inside, Pats was sitting on the end of an x-ray table talking to a Doctor Norman Jaffe. Michele was laying very still and quiet at the top of the table.

"Hi. What's happening?," I asked, handing her the screaming baby.

With a practiced motion, she unbuttoned her blouse and quickly quieted Patrick's protests with a well-filled breast.

"That's just what we're discussing," she said.

I looked at Norman Jaffe. He didn't look me in the eye.

136

"What's the problem?," I asked of anyone in the room who might be able to answer.

"Well, we're just not sure," Jaffe said in his measured British accent.

"What aren't we sure of, Doctor Jaffe?," I pressed.

"Were not sure of what it is we see," he stalled.

"What do you think you see, for Christ's sake?," I said, feeling my temperature starting to rise as this medicine man shuffle continued. "Can I have a straight answer, please."

"As I said, we're just not sure, as yet," he continued to fence with me.

"Doctor Jaffe, I'm trying very hard to be very patient with you. What do you THINK you see?," I demanded.

"Excuse me, one moment, please," he said, stepping out of room number three and into the clerk's area just a few feet away.

I turned toward Patsy and was about to start quizzing her on what had happened here this morning when I heard Jaffe say to the clerk, "Please call Doctor Filler and ask him to come over right away. He seems to be the only one here who can handle Mister Nolan."

Pats said that they had done the x-rays and the films showed a shadow in the back part of the brain that didn't appear normal. They had just finished with the brain scan and were unwilling to discuss it in any detail, electing, instead, to talk in vague generalities and to continue to say that they didn't know what they were seeing, but that they were seeing something unusual.

Jaffe returned to the room.

"Let's have a look at this brain scan. Maybe you can talk about it better if we see what you're looking at," I suggested, still pretty agitated.

"Doctor Filler will be right here. If we could just wait for a moment. I'd like to tell him what we see, first. I'm sure he will then be happy to discuss it with you in detail, but I want to consult with him before I say anything," Jaffe said.

"Bullshit! What the hell are we talking about here?"

At that moment, Michele started to experience another headache. She closed her eyes tightly and let out a soft, low whimper. Tears started to run down her cheeks and her mouth drew up in a frown of pain. I turned from Jaffe and put my hand on her head, trying to erase the pain from that tiny head.

I tried to comfort her as the pain built in that tiny head. "Easy, Baby. It'll be gone in just a second,"

Pats put out her free hand and touched Michele's thin leg.

"It hurts, Daddy. It really hurts bad," Michele said through the tears.

"I know, Honey. We're going to deal with that right away. Just try to relax. You know it hurts less when you just lay real still and don't move or talk or cry," I reminded her.

"I know, but it hurts real bad, Daddy," she said softly.

The pain was actually starting to ease. I could see the muscles in her face beginning to relax. In a few seconds she seemed to be free of the vice that gripped her delicate head in its jaws of iron.

"It's going away."

"I know. I'm glad. Now, just lay very still. We need to talk to Doctor Jaffe for a minute," I said as I wiped the big tear off of her pale cheek.

"Okay," she said quietly. She knew, even at that tender age, that she was in serious trouble.

Bob Filler must have run from his office to the other side of the hospital where we were. He was there, with us, in what seemed to be less than a couple of minutes.

"Hi. What's up, Norman?," he asked as he gave Patsy a quick hug around the shoulders and touched the top of Patrick's nursing head. Bob Filler loves the sight of babies and nurturing and love.

"I'd rather speak to you privately, if I may, Doctor Filler."

"Norman, you might just as well tell us all what you think. I'm just going to tell them what you tell me. So save some time and some energy and let's have it," he said firmly.

"Well, if you'd rather." Jaffe hated being placed in this, for him, very uncomfortable position by the Chief of Surgery.

"We have just completed the brain scan and there's a rather large area in the left occipital hemisphere that looks like it might be an abnormal mass," he said quietly, as though if he spoke softly we wouldn't hear what he really didn't want to tell us.

"Is this a tumor, we're seeing?," I asked.

"Yes, we think it is," he said, without looking at me.

"Why couldn't you have said that ten minutes ago?," I wanted to know.

Patsy raised her free hand to silence me. Giving her full attention to Jaffe she asked, "Is it the Wilm's, again?"

Norman Jaffe relaxed a little as he attempted to give her a more complete answer than he had offered up to now.

"We don't have any way of knowing just yet. Half of the people who experience a second incident of cancer develop the same cancer as they originally had and the other half are affected by a completely different cancer. It could be the Wilm's, although I'd think that would be highly unlikely since we have only seen four previous cases of Wilm's cranial metastasis in the past seventeen years here at the Jimmy Fund," he said.

"Only four?," I asked.

"In all the kids we've seen come through here in over seventeen years. While Wilm's is the second most common cancer in children, after Leukemia, it's very rare to have it move to the brain," Jaffe explained.

"What else could it be?," I asked.

"Another form of cancer, a benign tumor or some other type of growth."

"With the speed that this thing seems to be growing — I mean she didn't even have a headache three days ago — I'd say it's probably a Wilm's and she's just one of those super rare cases we seldom see. Let's have a look at the film, Norman," Bob said.

Now we were really crossing the line. We were being taken back to the viewing room where only the privileged are allowed to venture. It was as though we were being asked to join the generals in the war room.

"Michele, we're just going into the next room. Will you be okay here for a few minutes?," Patsy, who was still nursing Patrick, asked as she turned to reassure our daughter.

"Yes. It's okay, Mommy" she said.

"I'll stay with her," said the radiology technician, who had been in the room all the time, but who had remained silent and almost invisible during our discussion with the two doctors.

"Thanks," I said, patting her arm. She smiled at me, knowing that we were deeply concerned about a little girl who she knew was in terrible trouble. The technician was on the verge of tears, herself. Michele has the ability to touch people very quickly.

In the darkened room, with the walls of white, back-lighted viewing boxes, we looked at two small x-ray plates. We were joined by a senior surgical resident in the hospital's neurosurgical department, who had supervised the brain scans.

"These are from the brain scan. As you can see, there is this rather sizable dark area in this part of the brain," the young resident said, as he pointed to the black spot on an otherwise gray film. On the film was the outline — in about one-quarter size — of a left side view of Michele's head.

The other plate was from the front and you could see the same dark area on the left side of that scan.

"It's in the left rear, or motor sensory part of the brain. She is right handed, isn't she?," he asked.

"Yes," Patsy said.

"Well, from what we can tell from this study, it appears to be completely encapsulated and is not near the intelligence portion of the brain nor is it in the area where memory might be affected," he explained, maybe a little too eagerly.

"OK. So now we know what's causing the headaches. What the hell do we do about it?," I said, wanting him to cut right to the bottom line.

"Before we prescribe a course of treatment, we'd like to do the EEG. It might shed some more light on the problem," Norman Jaffe said.

"Fine. When do we do that?," I wanted to know.

"They're waiting for us, now," the resident said.

"I'll be in my office, if you need me," Bob Filler said. "I have several patients that I just walked out on. They're waiting for me to get back."

"Ran out on, is probably more like it," I said.

"Thanks, Bob, very much," Patsy said to him. He gave her a squeeze on the shoulder, smiled his "it's going to be okay" smile and slipped out the door.

I turned back to the surgical resident. "Is this something we operate on, right away?"

"I think the sooner, the better. It's probably growing as we speak. I don't know how much more pressure she can stand before the pain causes her to lose consciousness. It must be excruciatingly painful, given the size of it," he said.

"Are you prepared to do the surgery?," I asked him.

"Certainly," he said.

"Have you ever done this before?," I wanted to know.

"If this is a Wilm's, no one's ever done this before," he said quietly.

"What about the other four kids?," I asked for the first time, not really wanted to have the answer before now.

"They never made it to surgery. This type of cancer grows very fast," Norman Jaffe said.

"You mean that nobody has ever survived a Wilm's in the brain?," Patsy asked.

"Not that we know of. And we see more Wilm's tumor at the Jimmy Fund than any place else in the world," Jaffe assured us.

"Jesus, you'd better be real good," I said to the young resident.

"I'll do my best," he said in the confident tone of the young and eager.

I elected to go with Michele to the neurological department and stay with her for the EEG. It's a painless examine where they glue tiny electrodes onto her scalp and measure the electrical activity and patterns of electrical energy in her brain. It's a lot like an EKG measures electrical activity in the heart.

The EEG technician, at first, wasn't terribly pleased to have me there instead of out in the waiting room, but I didn't ask for her permission. I just stood by the table where Michele was laying, her head toward the technician and the monitor with it's delicate needles and long roll of graph paper. I could easily see into the technician's area as I was holding Michele's tiny hand. I could watch as the EEG needles recorded her delicate brain waves.

As the test began, I could see the needles wiggle as they traced the electrical activity inside Michele's head. In a few minutes one of the needles started to swing a wider arc from side to side.

"Oh, oh, look at that," said the technician, who was now more relaxed about my presence.

"Michele," I said, "you're about to have a headache, baby. Try to relax."

Sure enough, in just a second, her eyes squinted closed. Her tiny fingers squeezed my hand tightly. She emitted a low groan. I tried to reassure her that it would pass.

In seven or eight seconds, I saw the needles begin to return to the normal, smaller wiggles. I told her that the headache was on its way out. It would be gone in just a second. The technician smiled up at me. It looked like I had joined her team.

The EEG test continued for several minutes and Michele had three more headaches while it was being done. Each time I was able to caution her that it was coming and reassure her that it was going to stop, before she felt it ease up. It was an unforgettable experience for me to actually, graphically, watch my child have a series of brief, but very painful, headaches.

While Patrick was with Michele, I finished feeding the baby and took him with me to the admissions office to sign the papers, admitting Michele to Childrens Hospital for the third time in ten months. All of the clerks in the admissions office wanted to hold Patrick.

As I signed my name, I wondered just what we were going to do with Patrick. How was I going to be here with Michele and still tend to his needs, not the least of which was his need to nurse every few hours. It was going to be a difficult problem to solve. I really didn't know what we were going to do, but I knew we'd handle it — somehow.

When the EEG test was over, I called BZ and told the staff and Mel that I wasn't going to be there the rest of the day and maybe not tomorrow. We were not clear on the schedule of the proposed surgery and Michele was what was important, not a morning television program. There were other people at the station who could do the show. I had to do what I had to do, here at Childrens.

After an orderly and I had wheeled Michele up to her room on the seventh floor, I went down to see Bob Filler in his office.

"Hi. Got a minute?," I asked, sticking my head in the door to his office on the first floor of the hospital's clinical wing.

"Sure, come on in," he said, getting up and coming around the desk.

"Bob, what do we do about this new tumor?"

"We attack as quickly as possible. If we're not aggressive, it'll win, Patrick. And I know none of us wants to lose that baby now."

"Or ever."

"Or ever," he agreed.

"But do we just rush her down to the OR and chop in there?"

"If this is a Wilm's, and we all seem to agree now that Wilm's is the very best probability, we don't have much time. This stuff grows so fast you can almost watch it get bigger. Of course, that's one advantage we have over this type of cancer," he told me.

"Advantage? A swiftly growing cancer gives us an advantages? You're kidding?," I was terribly confused.

This cancer was growing so rapidly in the head of my little girl that her head might explode and Bob Filler was telling me that this gave us an advantage.

"You see, because it grows so fast, we can discover it much more quickly than one of the slower growing type of cancer. The slower growing ones can do all kinds of damage before we even know the patient is sick. This Wilm's tumor type shows up in a matter of days or weeks and we can attack before it spreads or does too much damage," he carefully and somewhat optimistically explained.

"How long has this stuff been growing in her brain, do you think?," I asked.

"Only a few days, weeks at the most. The tumor she had removed in L.A., the one that was the size of a grapefruit, had probably only been there for a couple of weeks. Less than a month I'm sure. Possibly only days, actually," he guessed.

"As it was, she hadn't showed any signs of being ill, until the night she fell," I reminded him.

"That's why it's so important to note any significant change in your child, even if there has been no loss of appetite, no fever or other symptoms. Sometimes this Wilm's stuff just drops out of the night and bites an innocent child, always without warning.

"Did you know that there have been cases of children being born with an active tumor?," he asked.

"No I didn't," I answered with some astonishment.

"Most cases are between birth and six years of age. The younger it develops the better the survival rate," he told me.

"Why do you suppose that is?," I wondered.

"We discover it sooner, I think. Mom is always touching, handling, watching a baby or a real small toddler. By the time they get to be five or six, they dress themselves and are more independent. We touch them less. It's usually discovered by Mom when she's dressing them or changing them," he said.

"Michele wasn't even sick and that damn thing was the size of a softball in her three year old body," I said.

"That's what I mean. It showed up before it has had time to run around doing a lot of other mischief. That's why we've been able, with an aggressive program of treatment and surgery, to reverse the odds on Wilm's survival. Fifteen years ago, when Doctor Farber started working on the problem here in the basement of Childrens Hospital, eighty-five out of a hundred kids who were diagnosed with a Wilm's tumor, died. Today, eighty-five out of a hundred patients live at least five years, many for a full, long life.

"This time around it just happens to be in a real tough place for Michele. Nobody has been able to deal with it as a cranial metastasis, mainly because it's so damn rare," he continued.

"So, no matter what we do, her chances are slim," I said.

"Well, let me explain the odds this way. The earlier it develops, the better the chances to survive. In Michele's case, she was three, right in the middle, so her chances were better that fifty-fifty. When it came back in her lungs five months later, her odds dropped to about twenty percent because that's what happens when it proves to be so resistant to treatment. Now, it's back for the third time and if it were say, in the other kidney or the liver or in the lungs, again, it would lower her odds to less than ten percent."

"But, it's not in her liver or lungs. It's growing in her brain," I reminded him.

"That means there are no odds. No one's ever survived this condition. But there have only been four cases in seventeen years, so we don't have a very big sample to gauge the odds of survival on, in all honesty," he explained, trying to be upbeat.

"Her odds may be zero, but I'll be damned if I'm going to give up on her. Now, who the hell does the surgery? I'm afraid I may have given that young resident the impression that it's his job. I don't know why. I guess I wasn't thinking too clearly at the time," I said, almost to myself.

"Don't worry about that, I'll speak to him. We have several people on the staff who are very good. Any one of them will do a good job," he assured me.

"Bob. Never mind that, we've got several good neurosurgeons', business. If it's your daughter, who the hell does it?" I asked him pointedly.

Without hesitation he said, "You go take care of your family. I'll speak to Larry Page about Michele. He'll be up to see her as soon as I can get him to look at the tests and the x-rays. He's a terrific surgeon and a terrific guy. You'll like him, I'm sure," he said, walking me to the door with his arm on my shoulder.

"Thanks, Bob. I'll never be able to repay the debt I'm building up with you."

142

I met up with Pats in the lobby. She had just finished the paperwork, admitting Michele.

I took Patrick from her and suggested that I go home, call Mom and ask her to return to New England, one more time.

I was also planning to get some clothes for Patrick and the other things we would need to keep him here in Boston as we took turns watching him in the lobby and comforting Michele on the seventh floor.

As yet, we didn't know what the next few days held in store for Michele or for us. I also had to arrange for one of the neighbors to watch after Teresa while we waited for Grandma Charlotte to come from California to take charge of things, again. I sure asked a lot of both our wonderful moms back in those stressful days.

Patsy got on the elevator and went to see Michele and Patrick the seventh and his father climbed into their Ford Mustang and went home to Sudbury.

The Reeds said that Teresa could stay with them until Mom came, in fact, they would be happy to pick Mom up at the airport for us.

Carol and David Reed are special people. I miss them sometimes. I hope they're well. A few years after Michele's surgery, they would lose their beautiful oldest daughter, Sherry. I was never quite able to repay their kindness to us when they suffered their terrible loss. I wish I could have been more help to them. Losing Sherry almost killed both of them. We were with them the night she died. It was just awful.

When I got home, I called Mom. She couldn't get here until the end of the week. I arranged for her ticket to be at the airport.

Then I called the office to tell them that I wouldn't be at the studio tomorrow. All of them, including Gladys, wished us the best. A wonderful group of people worked at WBZ-TV and WBZ radio during 1969.

The staff said not to worry, the show would be better without me. They were probably right about that.

Patrick and I were home about an hour when Charlie Austin walked in the front door, without knocking. I was fixing myself a sandwich.

"Hi, Charlie. Want something to eat?," I said as he walked over, kissed me and went down the hall towards the bedrooms.

"Nope."

Charlie can be a man of few words, even though he's one of the most respected television reporters in Boston, maybe in all of television news.

"How did you know I was home, Charlie?"

"I called the hospital and talked to Patsy after you called the station," he said disappearing down the hall.

"Where are you going?" No answer.

I got up and followed him as he turned into Patrick's nursery. He picked up what we used to call a diaper bag and began to pack Patrick's clothes into it.

"Pardon me, but what the hell do you think you're doing?"

"I'm taking the kid. You and Patsy have more than you need to deal with without having this little crumb grabber on your hands," he said with a note of finality.

"Charlie, you can't feed him. Patsy's the only one who can feed him. He's nursing, exclusively."

"Linda can feed him," he said with a smile that highlighted the gap between his two front teeth.

"She's got a new baby of her own to feed. She doesn't need another one. Besides, how is she going to feed them both?," I wanted to know.

"It's the old law of supply and demand, my friend. Linda called the doctor and he said that the more they drink, the more she'll make. It might be a little tight for them for the first day, but they'll both survive."

Charlie wasn't paying any attention to my protests. He was packing another bag with baby clothes.

When he finished emptying out Patrick's small chest of drawers, he picked up the bags, walked into the living room where Patrick was sleeping in his "infaseat" — a fore runner to the child car seat — picked him up and walked out the door.

"Don't worry about this little rug rat," he said. "Come get him when you get through this problem. And kiss Patsy for me."

With that, he took my six-week old baby boy out the door and left for Lexington, where the Austin clan lived. We wouldn't see Patrick for the next six days.

Shaking my head, I climbed back into the Mustang, this time alone, and went back to Childrens Hospital in Boston, worried now only about Michele. Thanks to Charlie & Linda Austin, the problem of what to do with Patrick was solved, at least until my Mom arrived to take charge of the household.

As I drove back to Childrens Hospital, I started to think about what lay ahead for us. I was very eager to meet Doctor Larry Page, neurosurgeon.

"I really don't want Michele to die, Dad,"
Teresa said to me, with big tears rolling down her face.
"I don't want her to die either, baby."
"Do you know why I mostly don't want her to die?"
"No, I don't," I told her, kissing away a tear.
"Cause if Michele dies, Patrick will never,
ever get to know his big sister," she sobbed.

Chapter Nine

"Hi, I'm Larry Page!"

When I got back to Childrens Hospital, Patsy was upstairs with a very quiet Michele, who was experiencing another of her headaches — or as the doctors called them, abnormal cerebral events.

By now the pressure in her eyes was so severe that she was only slightly aware of what was going on around her. She had all she could do just to concentrate on dealing with the pain each time that thing in her head increased the pressure on her brain. It was decided not to administer any pain medication until the neurosurgeon had been up to personally examine her.

A few minutes after I arrived in Michele's room, Pasty asked me who was in the lobby with Patrick.

"Patrick's not in the lobby."

"He's probably screaming his head off for something to eat, by now. It's been four hours since he nursed. I'm about to burst. Where is he?"

Patsy's mammary glands were filled to the brim with warm milk. She wanted a donor just as much as she surmised Patrick wanted a donation.

"He's not here," I said calmly.

"What do you mean he's not here?"

"I sold him."

"Will you please just tell me what you've done with our child?"

She was about through playing this game.

"I told you. I sold him... to Charlie and Linda."

"Charlie and Linda have him? Patrick, how can you ask Linda to take care of Patrick? She has a new baby of her own to deal with," she scolded me, thinking that I had asked Linda to take Patrick.

"Believe me, Babe, I didn't have anything to say about it. After Charlie talked to you on the phone, here, he drove out to Sudbury, packed Patrick's clothes in a suitcase and walked out with the kid under his arm. He didn't even ask me to open the door for him. He took the kid and left. He did send you a kiss."

"But how are the Austins going to feed him?"

"Charlie barely said three words to me, but he did say something about the laws of supply and demand."

"Oh my God. Linda's going to try to feed them both."

A soft voice from the bed interrupted us. "Mommy, it hurts again."

"Try to relax, Michele. Remember, at home, when you just laid down on the floor and didn't move? It didn't hurt as bad, did it?"

"No."

"It'll pass in a second, Honey," Pats said, stroking Michele's head as gently as she possibly could. She was using the Magic Mother fingers, trying to ease the pain in her baby.

It was very difficult to watch as our tiny child endured wave after wave of ever greater pain from those headaches.

It wasn't as though she had been free of pain for the past ten months. Although the other occurrences had been painful for Michele, the pain had quickly gone away a few days after each surgery. But this time, the intense pain was literally blinding our child as it continued to intensify.

A few minutes after I arrived, a tall, lean stranger with premature flecks of gray sprinkled throughout his dark hair appeared. He was slightly hunched and seemed relaxed as he walked into Michele's room.

"Hi, there. I'm Larry Page," he said casually, with just the slight hint of a Dixie accent in his voice.

His face was a very pleasant one, with bright blue eyes and a friendly grin. He was a handsome man, with a calm, easy manner about him.

"Nice to meet you," I said as we shook hands.

"Mrs. Nolan."

"It's Patsy."

"OK, Patsy. Bob Filler asked me to have a look at Michele."

One of the first things I noticed about Larry Page was that he really looked at you when he spoke to you or when you spoke to him. For Larry, eye contact was important.

As he gently examined her, he talked directly to Michele. He asked his questions of her, not about her, through us.

So often when a small child is involved, a doctor will interview the parents about how the child feels, as though the child were not in the room.

Larry asked Michele how often the pain begins. (right after it stops), when it did start — what part of her head hurt first. (the top, toward the back). He wanted to know if her eyes hurt when the headache came. (they did). He wanted to know if anything else hurts, tummy, chest, arms, anything. (they didn't).

I think, in an attempt to assess just how much the tumor may have affected her mental capacities, he casually said, "Michele, I understand your Momma's a nurse."

"No. She isn't."

A puzzled look came on Larry's face for a split second, before Michele finished her answer.

"She used to be a nurse, but now she's just a Mommy."

"Well," said Larry, with a smile, "so much for any confusion or inability to reason."

Patsy and I could only return Larry's smile, chuckle softly and shake our heads in amazement.

After Larry was through looking at Michele, he walked us out into the hallway. I assured Michele that we weren't going far and that we'd be right back.

Michele's room was at the end of the hall. There was a certain degree of privacy just outside the door, in a little alcove that held a large window. Out that window I could see the Peter Bent Brigham Hospital where Larry did most of his work. The Brigham was, like the Jimmy Fund, connected to Childrens by a series of enclosed bridges. How many people, I wondered as I looked out that window, are there over in that big, gray building, hurting as much as I am right now?

How many husbands, wives, sons, daughters or lovers are standing in a white hallway getting bad news about a loved one from a man in a white coat?

Now, I thought, here comes our bad news.

"I've just looked at the EEG, the x-rays and the brain scan and have examined the results of her blood tests," Larry was saying.

"We're dealing with a fairly large tumor in the back left side of her brain," he said, touching the back of his own head with long, strong fingers.

"We don't know, at this time, if it's a benign or a malignant tumor. If it is malignant we have no way of knowing, yet, if it's a Wilm's. It may be another, completely different, type of malignancy. I strongly suspect that it's a Wilm's however. What I do know is this, it should be removed as quickly as possible."

"Do you think you can remove it?," Patsy asked.

"Yes, but we can't operate on that little girl until we've reduced, and I mean seriously reduced, the swelling and the pressure that the tumor is causing. I really can't understand why she's not in a coma or at the very least, unconscious with all the pressure she has in there. That's one tough little kid ya'll have got in there. The pressure on her brain is tremendous."

"What do you suggest we do?"

"I've ordered a series of things to be done right away. First, we'll give her some steroids to try to reduce the swelling. Steroids, as you know, tend to reduce the symptoms: the swelling, the inflammation and so forth, but they don't cure or heal anything. What they do — sometimes — is mask the things that get in the way of our being able to fix things."

Pats and I quietly listened as this gentle young surgeon explained to us what he saw as our best course of action for Michele. I can't tell you how comforting it was to hear him carefully explain the steps he planned to take in treating Michele. As I listened to him, I began to believe that he could actually save her life.

"So, the first thing we have to do is work on getting the pressure down, but," he continued, "we've also got to try to strike a balance here. We need to take the time to reduce the swelling and the pressure, but not too much time. If it is another Wilm's, you know that they grow very rapidly. Time is also our enemy."

"Does she really have a chance?," Patsy asked directly. "Norman Jaffe says that nobody's ever survived a Wilm's tumor in the brain."

"Someone will, one day and it might as well be Michele and it might as well be now. She's still alive, so, naturally I think we still have a chance of being successful."

147

Instantly it seemed, both Patsy and I clearly understood Larry's attitude about what looked like insurmountable odds. As long as she was still alive, she still had a chance to survive. We knew that Larry Page wasn't the kind of guy who gave in to his enemy easily. And death was this man's daily foe.

"How long do you think we have, realistically, to get the pressure down and do the surgery?," I asked.

"Only a few days, really. I'd think that we're looking at surgery on Thursday, Friday at the latest. Fortunately, for her, we've identified the problem at what looks like the earliest possible stage. That, at least, is in her favor. And Michele seems to be a real fighter to me," he said with a grin.

"She's tough as nails, just like her Mom," I told him as I gently hugged the lady who once had been a nurse, but who was now just Michele's marvelous Mommy.

"There are some folks around here who think you two are the tough ones. I've talked to a dozen people so far about you and most of them think you're concerned, involved, terrific parents. But there are some others who think you're pretty hard to deal with. I don't think I've ever heard such widely conflicting opinions of two people before in my life."

I looked at him calmly, "That doesn't surprise me in the least. What do you think?"

"Oh, we've just met. But I'm putting my money on the ones who think you're concerned and involved. We'll just have to see how it goes."

"That's fair," I said.

Patsy squeezed my hand and forced a smile up at me.

"What do we do for the next three days?," Patsy asked.

"Just try to keep her quiet and as comfortable as you can 'til we can get some of that pressure relieved. I think when we get some of the swelling down she'll be a lot more comfortable."

"I'm pleased that you're as up front with us as you've been. We both deeply appreciate that," Patsy told him.

"From what I've heard, I don't have much chance to be anything else with you two," he grinned.

"You've talked to Norman Jaffe, have you?"

"Dr. Jaffe's very concerned about your daughter. It's just that he's just been trained in England and he finds it difficult to step through the barrier which he's built around himself. He's really a fine physician," Larry said.

"I never questioned his medical credentials nor his medical skills. I just think he needs to work a little on his communication skills," I responded.

"By the way, Dr. Jaffe thinks you're both very fine parents. He doesn't fault your concern, he just wishes that you weren't quite so involved in every detail of Michele's treatment," Larry said.

"Sorry, can't go back. We've been too badly burned by you guys," I told him.

"Maybe you should tell me about that."

I gave him the abbreviated version of Morton Woolley's act the first time around.

"I'll try to do better, but maybe there were extenuating circum ..."

I broke him off by saying, "I don't give a damn."

"I'm sure you don't. I think I'll look in on Michele, again, and then run along. I'll be back a little later to see how the cortisone is affecting the pressure."

The next three days were devoted to reducing the symptoms of the disease. The steroids reduced the swelling, which in turned eased the pain. While Michele was still experiencing periodic headaches, she did seem to be a lot more comfortable, spending most of the day dozing.

At times, she seemed more restless than at other times. She still complained when a headache started, but she wasn't having any more of those horrible, blinding episodes.

Patrick was spending mornings at the studio, producing his television program, and his afternoons at the hospital, helping me look after Michele.

On Wednesday, two medical students came in to start an IV in Michele's arm. They spent several minutes washing and preparing Michele's thin limb, tying the tourniquet around it and looking for a good vein. They asked her to make a fist — which she did — and they slapped at her skin, as they tried to raise a vein, into which they wanted to insert the needle.

I looked at Patrick and Patrick looked at me and I guess we both thought, maybe one of them was born with the touch. We would rather have had an experienced IV nurse start the IV, but maybe one of these guys did have the talent.

The first guy pushed the needle against Michele's skin, then through the skin, and he actually did that part rather well.

But when the sharp needle entered the vein, he didn't stop. He kept right on going until he had pushed the needle right out the other side of the vein. Seeing that the syringe was not filling with blood, he nervously looked at his companion. Even I know you don't draw blood from muscle tissue.

Next he pulled back on the needle, not just until it was back in the vein, but clear out of her arm. The spot where he'd stabbed her with the needle started to bleed.

"She's really got tiny veins," he said, in his own defense.

Then he poked the needle in again, trying to hit the vein which was turning purple and bulging up through her paper thin skin at him. This time the needle pushed off the vein as he drove it deep into her tiny arm.

"Missed, again."

"Here," said the other guy, "Let me try."

"No, let's not," Patrick said firmly.

"I'm sorry?," said the first guy.

"That's it, guys. You two need to go somewhere and practice on each other, 'cause you're through practicing on Michele."

For a second or two, nobody moved. There was an embarrassed air of tension in the room.

"I'm sorry, Sir, but I'll have to ask you and your wife to leave the room," one of them said, trying desperately to salvage a little of their newly developing medical dignity and assertive physicians manner.

"Sorry, but that's not going to happen. And this effort of yours to start an IV is over," Patrick told them in no uncertain terms.

"Sir, I know you're upset, but we have a job to do here and you're not helping much. It might be better if you stepped out of the room for a minute. This will only take a minute to complete."

"The only thing I'm going to let you two do is *leave* this room," Patrick said, even more firmly.

"We were sent in to start this IV and while I'm sorry that it's not going as well as you'd like, it's something we have to do."

"Wrong! Neither one of you is going to touch my daughter again. What you are going to do is leave this room and I mean both of you and I mean right now, without another word," Patrick said calmly, but with an unmistakable edge of steel in his voice.

Both young medical students looked at each other, then at me, then they looked at Patrick and then, without a word, they put down the equipment they were holding and left Michele's room. They, of course, really didn't have any other option.

"I'll bet you just made the top ten on both of their pain in the butt lists," I said.

"Happy to be listed," Patrick said.

"Pats, will you please go call Bob Filler? Tell him that he'd better do something about his medical students before one of them gets hurt. I'll stay here with Michele to see that those two guys don't try to sneak back in here while you're gone and attack her again."

Patrick was really upset with those two clumsy fools. I was too. I've never seen, in all my years in training and in nursing, two more inept practitioners with a needle. Granted, starting an IV is an acquired skill, but those two were just completely unskilled. As Patrick had suggested to them, they needed to practice on each other a little more.

I went out to the desk to call Dr. Filler's office. The nurse asked me if she could do anything for me. The nurse had probably gotten an ear full from the two medical students when they returned from Michele's room.

"No, I just need to talk to Dr. Filler, please."

She dialed the number and handed me the phone.

When Bob came on the phone. I told him that a couple of his students had botched up an IV and that we needed his help. He said he'd be right up.

When Bob stepped off of the elevator, I was waiting for him.

He said, "Let's get an IV tray."

"I have everything we need in Michele's room."

"Patrick threw them out, did he?"

"He certainly did," I told him.

"Do they need emergency care?," he asked, half in jest and half seriously.

"I don't think they'll ever be quite the same, but they're not bleeding. Although they probably should be," I said.

In a matter of minutes, Bob and I had the IV started and running fine in Michele's arm. He asked me to walk back down to the nurse's station with him.

As he was charting the fact that the IV was, indeed, now running properly, he said to the nurse behind the counter, "Nurse, may I have a red magic marker, please?"

"Certainly, Doctor Filler," she said, reaching into a nearby drawer.

"Here you are."

"Thank you."

Right across the top of Michele's chart, in letters about three inches high, he wrote, "NO MED STUDENTS!," with the magic marker. Then he carefully underlined each word and handed the chart and the marker back to the nurse.

"Please be sure that all medical students remain out of Michele Nolan's room, unless they're escorted by either Dr. Page or myself," he instructed.

"Of course, Doctor. Is there a problem?"

"Not now," I said, as I smiled at Bob.

Bob smiled back, as he shook his head at the nurse, telling her everything was fine, that the IV was running, but that she should check it in a few minutes.

I walked toward the elevator with Bob, thanking him for being there for us.

As he took my hands in his he reminded me that he had a certain stake in Michele's recovery, too.

"One of the reasons I selected pediatric surgery after my residency is that most of my patients get well, Patsy. I don't lose too many. I really like that. I don't want to lose Michele."

He paused then said, "Nor do I want to lose her father."

Bob Filler is a very wise man.

"Let me know if I can do anything else," he said.

"Thanks, I will."

When I told him about it, Patrick just loved the order Bob had written on the front of Michele's chart in red marker.

The next few days dragged by as the steroids did what they could to get Michele ready for surgery. Between the reduced pressure and the pain medication she was getting, Michele was somewhat more comfortable. Her head hurt all the time now, but it was more of a dull ache then the razor sharp, excruciating pain that she'd experienced on Monday.

On Thursday afternoon Larry Page came in and put his arm around my shoulders.

"Patsy, we do it tomorrow morning or we don't do it. We're not going to get her any better than she is, right now. If we wait any longer, it will start to grow and our control will go down hill on us and we'll be unable to even attempt surgery."

Smiling, and using a Star Trek analogy, Larry said, "So, first thing in the morning we'll try to go where no man has gone before," he said, with a reassuring smile and the strong confidence that made both Patrick and I feel just a little better.

"Do you have any questions?," Larry asked as he was about to leave.

I locked my eyes on his for a few seconds before I said calmly but seriously, "Yes. Yes, I have a thousand questions, Larry. I just don't know what they are. But you do."

He paused a moment, carefully thinking about what I'd just said to him.

"Of course you have. Well, I'll sure try to give you the answers, even if you don't know the questions," he said, almost tenderly.

"That's exactly what we want, Dr. Page. That's what we both want," Patsy said, putting her arm on my shoulder.

Dr. Larry Page, surely one of the world's most gifted neurosurgeon, was able to examine what I had said to him about that horrible routine medical question, *do you have any questions*, and alter his behavior. Even after eight years as a neurosurgical resident, he was able to learn from a parent.

A few days later Larry told me that he didn't think he would ever again ask anyone that question. He should know, he said, that everyone has lots of questions at a time like this, but of course they don't know what the questions are. After all, he said, he had been a neurosurgical resident for eight years before he thought he even knew some of the questions, much less any of the answers.

Dr. Larry Page has a healthy ego — as all good surgeons must surely have to perform the work they perform — but he doesn't let his ego get in the way of having a terrific bedside manner or in the way of his continuing education as a physician. Larry is wise enough to know that he can actually learn something new from his patients or their family, from time to time. Larry Page is a very special physician and a very special person.

On the day of Michele's brain surgery, Larry said something that turned out to be immensely important. Nothing could have prepared us for the importance of what he said to us that day, but it was one of the most thoughtful things anyone has ever said to me. It had a tremendous impact on reducing our fears. It also had a wonderfully calming effect on both of us.

Larry instinctively knew that we were extremely concerned about tomorrow's delicate brain surgery. Brain surgery is a major risk for most folks, but for Michele, in her condition, he knew that we were exceptionally worried that she might not survive the procedure. He took my hand and put his other hand on Patrick's arm as we sat together outside Michele's room.

"Tomorrow," Larry said, "I want both of you to keep one thing in mind, all day. The surgery, while certainly both major in scope and very serious in nature, is of absolutely no risk to Michele, even though this particular tumor has never been successfully removed before."

For just a second, I couldn't believe that I had actually heard Larry say what he had just said to us. Had he actually said that the surgery was without any risk to Michele?

Patrick had a very puzzled expression on his face as he asked, "What the hell are you talking about, Larry? You're going to saw a three inch hole in the top of a four year old child's head and you're telling us that there's no risk involved?"

"That's exactly what I'm telling you. The surgery is no risk to Michele. None, what so ever. The tumor is killing her. If we do nothing, she'll be dead in a few days. We all recognize that as a fact. Tomorrow, if she dies on the operating table, all she's lost is a few days of terrible pain. The surgery will not have taken her life because it's the tumor that's responsible for killing her."

"I never thought of it that way before, but you're right," I said.

152

"Our job tomorrow is to remove the tumor, if we can, and not to let the cancer have its way. But, remember, the cancer is what's putting her at risk, not the surgery," Larry said.

"Do you think her chances tomorrow are any better than zero?," Patrick asked.

"If we don't do the surgery, we know her chances are absolutely zero. As I said, she'll be gone within a few days — weeks, certainly. Remember, this is a very rare opportunity. None of the other kids that had this happen to them even got to the OR. This time we think we have a slim chance of doing something about it, because we're seeing it at such a very early stage."

Was he trying to plant an excuse for what might be a failure in the morning?

No. What Larry was doing was extremely thoughtful and very considerate. He was trying to take away as much of our anxiety about the surgery as he could by placing the real threat to Michele's life — that growing tumor in her brain — in the proper perspective. The surgery — complicated, difficult and delicate as it was going to be was not to be feared. The tumor was Michele's only enemy, not Larry's scalpel.

"Well, I guess that puts tomorrow in a completely different light. Silly me, I was worried sick about major brain surgery on our baby," Patrick said as he listened carefully to Larry.

While he was making a dark joke about tomorrow, Patrick deeply appreciated what Larry had just done for us. So did I.

"And remember this, too, about tomorrow. The longer it takes, the better for Michele, the better for all of us. So don't start worrying if we're not back down here in four or five or even six hours. The worst thing we could do tomorrow is rush. This is, after all, Michele's only chance. We have to do it right," he said.

"I don't have anything else on my calendar for tomorrow. I'm not playing cards tomorrow night, I don't have guests coming for dinner. I'm not taking any calls from my stockbroker. Tomorrow, the only thing I have to do is take that thing out of Michele's head, so we won't be in any hurry," Larry told us as we stood there beside Michele's bed.

Larry, by providing more than just his wonderful surgical skills, had helped us focus on what was really important. He had shown us what was, in fact, Michele's reality. The rapidly growing tumor was killing her, that was an absolute fact. The surgery couldn't kill her. The only thing that surgery could possibly do tomorrow would be to make her better. It couldn't kill her.

Then Patrick put his hand on Larry's hand and said to him softly, with tears in his eyes, "Thank you. But will you remember something for us tomorrow? If this thing is beyond doing, don't send us back a cantaloupe. If it can't be removed, without destroying Michele, then don't take it out."

Here we were, on the brink of losing our daughter, and Patrick wanted Larry to fully understand that we had both accepted her death as the most likely result for tomorrow's surgery. Of course, we hadn't given up hope that she would survive — mainly because Michele had not given up hope — but we knew that the odds of her being the first to survive what none before had survived were very, very slim. Patrick just didn't want there to be any doubt in Larry's mind that we had completely come to terms with the probability that, this time, the cancer might actually win. If nothing could be done to reverse that, Patrick told him, "Do nothing."

Of course, I agreed completely.

"I won't destroy her, no matter what we find tomorrow," Larry said softly as he put his other hand on Patrick's shoulder and looked deeply into his eyes. "I won't do that to her, I promise."

We all just stood there silently for a moment. It was a moment of intense feelings.

"Thanks!," Patrick said. "Thanks a lot."

Then he reached over and carefully and lovingly wiped a tear from my cheek.

"Michele, I've got something to tell you," I said quietly as I sat holding her hand.

She was so tiny and so frail and so helpless. Gone was the puck that had been there throughout the other two surgeries and all the painful radiation and terrible chemotherapy treatments. Here instead was a fragile four year old child who might only be days, or even hours, away from the end of her struggle. I was a little frightened as I sat there because she seemed, for the first time, to be so nearly out of fight. The painful headaches and the terrible pressure that was building in her brain were extracting a terrible toll from our baby daughter.

"Shelly, Doctor Page says he's going to take away your headache tomorrow."

"Good."

"But I have to tell you something. To do that, they're going to have to cut off all your hair. When you wake up after the surgery, all your hair will be gone," I said.

"Will it grow back?"

"Yes."

"Will my headache be gone, too?," she asked me.

"Yes. One way or the other, I promise, the headache will be gone," I said.

"Then they can cut off my hair," she said with all the pragmatism of a general going into battle knowing he's going to lose some men, but also knowing that if he doesn't engage the enemy in this battle he's going to lose the war.

"I just didn't want you to be worried about your hair when you woke up tomorrow after the operation."

"Why can't they take out the headache now?," she wanted to know.

She was so tired of all the IVs, the medication, the hospital, the doctors, the nurses and, of course, the pain.

"Well, they have to get a good night's sleep and so do you," I said, trying to comfort her in her impatience.

"But it really hurts, Daddy," she said. A single tear appearing in the corner of her eye as her mouth twisted into a soft sob.

"I know it does, Baby. I wish I could reach right in there and take out that damn headache, but we'll just have to be brave and wait for morning."

154

With huge tears in her eyes, Michele looked deeply into my eyes and asked, "Is Doctor Grayhair really going to take away my headache?"

One of the only bright spots in the past week had been when Michele had decided that Dr. Larry Page would be called, now and forever more, Doctor Grayhair.

"Yes. Doctor Grayhair is going to take out the headache tomorrow, before breakfast," I told her.

"Good!," she said with a note of finality.

I've always known when we had come to the end of one of our little talks. I kissed away a tear or two and went out into the hallway to shed a few of my own. Michele's father was very scared of what tomorrow might bring.

That night we drove home in almost complete silence. There really wasn't much more to say. We each knew what tomorrow meant. The prospect of continuing on, without Michele, wasn't a subject we really wanted to discuss right then. It wasn't something that either of us had ever really visualized, I don't think. At a time like this, your mind has all it can do to just keep up with the events as they unfold before you.

We had the strength we needed from each other. Our friends — even the very new ones — and our family were all terrific with their love and support, but it was Patsy's strength that I needed during this difficult time. I'd have been sunk without her quiet strength and wonderful confidence.

That night, when we went to bed, Patsy said that she wanted to make love to me.

"I need to be as close to you as I can get," she said through the tears.

Except for maybe the day we welcomed Patrick into the world, we were as close that night as two people could possible be to one another. That night, I too, needed desperately, to be that close to my partner.

The next morning, Friday, August 22, 1969, we were up early and at the hospital before they wheeled her down that long, cold hallway and through those electric swinging doors with the big sign on them that says, Surgery — No Admittance.

"Remember," Larry had said earlier that morning in her room, "It's going to be a while. We aren't going to be in any hurry today."

Michele had already had her pre-op sedative, so she was pretty groggy, but she did ask Patrick, one last time, if her headache was going to be gone when she woke up.

"I promise. The headache will be all gone when you wake up, Shelly," he told her as the doors swung opened and that tiny, brave little kid rolled in to face the toughest challenge she would ever face.

As she entered the operating suite in the basement of Childrens Hospital which would be today's arena for this life and death encounter, we knew that Michele was on her way to meet the enemy. We also knew that this afternoon only one of them would be coming back from that deadly meeting. Before the late summer sun would set, one of them would claim victory.

I don't believe there's another feeling in the world which is quite as desperate or as traumatic a feeling to me as standing there, outside those electric doors, watching your child being wheeled in to surgery and not be allowed to follow. It is a terrible feeling. Each time it's happened, my stomach is twisted into a tight, painful knot. The fear and anxiety are so enormous. You stand there and watch that final departure, knowing that it may well be the last time you'll see your child alive. For me, there's no getting used to that awful feeling. I know Patrick hated that feeling, too. But I don't think it affected him as deeply as it did me. At least I hope it didn't.

As the day, and the operation, dragged by, we had a steady stream of visitors. A couple of our favorite nurses from the Jimmy Fund came over on their lunch hour, just to hold our hands. One of them went up to the OR and looked through the glass windows to see if they were still working. She came back to report that they were still busy in their glass cage.

Bob Filler stopped by, at least three times, to give us an update.

"I just looked in and Larry gave me the thumbs up sign. I guess that's good news," he said.

Bob couldn't go in the room and ask how things were going because Michele's operating room was sealed, to prevent any contamination from entering the room as a hitchhiker. During most operations, only those who are going to actually handle the instruments or touch the sterile field are scrubbed and wearing sterile gloves. In this intercranial procedure, everyone who was going to be in the operating room, no matter what their job, had scrubbed. Once everyone went in, they locked the door, nobody came out — unless they stayed out — and no one entered until the procedure was over. You'd better plan your visits to the bathroom accordingly.

The nurse assigned to parents with children in surgery made sure she always knew where we were at all times that day.

This August day was a lovely, late summer day in New England. Patrick and I spend a lot of our time out in the beautiful flower garden that nestles between the towers of Childrens Hospital, just behind the cafeteria.

The garden at Childrens was donated, and maintained, by a woman who had, years before, lost her only two children to a serious illness.

Maida Pringle was from a very rich, prominent Boston family, but money couldn't save her baby girls. Even so, Mrs. Pringle was a very generous donor to Childrens Hospital over the years.

Mrs. Pringle frequently visited the hospital, helping out, as so many other wonderful ladies in Boston still do, as volunteers with the children. A group of very loving, gentle women, they read to the kids, tell them stories and are a very special group of Visiting Grandmothers. Many parents, whose children have been treated at Childrens Hospital, owe this marvelous group of ladies a great, unpayable, debt. I know we owe them more than we could ever repay.

One day, years before our Michele was even born, Mrs. Pringle walked out the back door of the cafeteria with the hospital administrator.

Looking at the empty area behind the new wing she asked, "What are you going to build out here?"

"This is going to be the doctor's parking lot, Mrs. Pringle."

"This should be a garden, for the children," she said, flatly.

"Yes," the administrator agreed, "It should be. But with the cost of the new building, we simply can't afford to build a garden here."

"Well, I certainly can afford to build it," she said.

And build it she did.

Not only did she pay to have a magnificent garden built, with bushes, trees, flowers and hedges, but she had them place some strategic benches in secluded areas of the garden for privacy and for crying.

The garden also had wide walkways for wheelchairs and carts. Mrs. Pringle lovingly supervised every detail of the garden's layout and construction. They say she selected each plant and each shrub personally.

After it was built, she continued to pay for it's maintenance. A trust fund which she left for that purpose maintains that lovely garden to this day.

Once, while Michele was in the hospital, I caught a brief glimpse of Mrs. Pringle. She was quite along in years by the time I saw her, but she was still coming to Childrens every week, with her two silver handled canes, giving gentle instructions to the three full time gardeners who cared for the flowers and the trees and the shrubs in the garden.

Mrs. Pringle had stone figures of small animals scattered throughout the garden. In one corner of the garden was a bear. Several rabbits peeked around the corner of a hedge. A tiny fawn, a fox, a boy and his dog, a turtle and several others were there for the children's pleasure. From time to time, Mrs. Pringle had the gardeners rearrange the location of the animals so that the garden always had a fresh look for the children.

This beautiful, restful garden was one of the most wonderful gifts anyone has ever given to a hospital. It continues to give thousands of parents and their children, a world of pleasure and joy. The garden at Childrens offers a quiet comfort to people. They find it so very peaceful, right there in the middle of an otherwise cold, sterile, hospital environment.

Thanks, Maida Pringle, from all of us who've found peace in your lovely garden. Thanks, a million.

As Patsy and I waited in Maida Pringle's garden, I thought about the toughest call I would have to make as soon as we knew the results of the surgery. I had to call and talk to our Charlie.

Teresa had come to me the day Michele went back in the hospital and asked me, point blank, "Dad, is Michele going to die?"

This was one of the most difficult conversations I ever had with one of my children. Here I was, not ready to come to terms with Michele's possible — if not probable — death, myself and I was being asked to help a seven year old face it.

"I don't know, Honey. She's real sick, this time, so I can't promise you that she won't die."

"I really don't want Michele to die, Dad," she said, with big tears rolling down her face.

As I kissed away the tears I said, "I don't either, Charlie."

"Do you know why I mostly don't want her to die, Dad?,"

"No, I don't," I said.

"Cause if she dies, Patrick will never, ever get to know his big sister," she sobbed.

"Well, I'm sure glad Patrick has you. You are about the best big sister anyone could possible have. Michele and Patrick are both very lucky."

She just put her arms around my neck and cried softly into my shoulder for several minutes. It was a moment I will never forget. It was a moment of great sadness, but it was also a moment of great tenderness between me and my oldest daughter. It was a moment filled with love, hope and very deep, wonderful feelings.

When she had stopped sobbing, she forced me to promise that as soon as the operation was over I'd call her — no matter what. I told her that I would.

I told her she'd better go directly to the Reeds after school to wait for my call there.

As we sat in Mrs. Pringle's garden that afternoon, I knew Charlie would be sitting there in the living room at Carol and David's, right next to the telephone, waiting for it to ring.

Teresa is a terrific big sister. Anyone who knows my sister will tell you that she's capable of great love. During the times when everyone in the family was worried about me, completely consumed with my surgeries, my treatments and my health, Teresa never once demanded attention. Never once did she act out any feelings of hostility toward me or my illness, demanding the spotlight for herself. She was content to be my big sister.

She always waited for me when I couldn't keep up. She always looked out for me when we played with other children. She was never the least bit jealous of the gifts I got from strangers nor jealous of the attention that was paid to me when I was sick.

My sister, Teresa, was, and is, a terrific big sister. Not only did she have to take a back seat to me and my troubles when I was sick, but just when she thought she might get some equal time, along came our baby brother, Patrick.

Born at home, the only boy, Patrick attracted a lot of attention to himself from friends and family. Grandma Charlotte even called him "His Majesty."

Here was Teresa, the first born and the first Nolan grandchild, relegated to third place by a sister with cancer and a new baby brother who was born at home.

I was an adult before I could fully appreciate how well she had behaved during the years when I was sick. I love my sister, Teresa, very, very much.

I, of course, remember very little about that long day in 1969 when Doctor Grayhair was adding to his growing reputation as a great surgeon. I spent the day sleeping. I do remember the bright lights in the operating room when they wheeled me in. I remember the faces of the doctors and the nurses, all hidden behind those little green masks. I remember Doctor Grayhair telling me that everything was going to be all right and I remember hearing him say that it was time for me to go to sleep. And, of course, I remember those awful headaches that just wouldn't go away.

As the day wore on, several people from the studio came by to visit us in the garden. Charlie Austin stopped by for a few minutes. Connie,

Patrick's production assistant, made a stop in the garden. Connie was a bright spot on most days. She had a delightful, disarming sense of humor. I don't remember who else came by, but I know there were others. They all helped a lot, just being there with us for a few minutes, showing us that they cared.

Most of the day, however, Patrick and I spent by ourselves, walking, sitting and holding hands in Mrs. Pringle's beautiful garden. We needed this peaceful, quiet garden to wait for the news we were so anxious to hear, yet, at the same time, dreaded so fiercely to hear.

Just as Larry had predicted, Friday turned out to be a very long day. The operation went on for over eight hours, but Maida Pringle's garden was a very peaceful place for two scared young parents to wait while magic was being performed upstairs.

Just before five in the afternoon, our special nurse — the one assigned to the parents of kids in surgery — walked quickly into the garden, looked around to find us and came directly to the bench where we were sitting.

"They just called from the OR. They're closing. Dr. Page said he would be on his way to see you in just a couple of minutes."

"Does he want to meet us in the parent's room?," Patrick asked.

"Yes. I'll take you there now," the nurse said.

"That's fine. We know where it is, thanks," he said.

"Of course."

Trying to be as positive as she could, without giving us any false hopes, the nurse said, "I feel things must have gone well. It's been such a long day for you, but sometimes, that's really good news."

"He told us that if it was going well it would take a while. We weren't looking for a one hour operation," I said, as the three of us walked toward the door that would lead us to that quiet, comfortable parent's room just off the lobby. The room where parents get good news and where parents get bad news.

We were there for only a few minutes when the door opened and a tall, thin, slightly hunched young surgeon walked in. We both stood up.

"She's just fine," were the first words out of his mouth as he came toward us, still wearing the green pants and scrub shirt of the OR.

"And I'm that high off the ground." He indicated his joy by holding out his hand about three feet above the floor.

"We did something today that no one's ever done."

Larry Page was elated. Here was a man who had just spent an entire day inside the brain of a four year old baby and he looked like he'd just won a million dollars in the lottery.

"Now, sit down. Let me tell you what we did," he said.

Patsy and I hugged each other and then we both reached out to Larry. We just had to make physical contact with this gifted physician. For us, shaking hands was out of the question, so we just hugged him. He hugged us right back.

"She's doing just great. As I said before the operation, that's one tough little gal you've got there. However, I really had no idea just how tough she was until today. Today, she had to be tough."

Calmly he explained how he and Michele had spent the day.

When they got Michele anesthetized, the pressure in her head still remained too high to open the skull without risking serious — and irreparable damage — to her brain. The brain could just explode if they opened her skull with that much pressure built up inside. While the steroids had helped some, they hadn't been strong enough weapons in this battle.

In the OR they administered a series of diuretic drugs to drastically reduce the fluids in Michele's entire system, but the pressure still remained too high to continue the operation.

Finally, they tapped her spinal column and drained out all of her spinal fluid. Michele was now in a very dangerous position. One mistake, one unfortunate jar to the table, could be fatal for her. But, as Larry had told us, the operation wasn't going to kill her. If she died, it would be the tumor that killed her. That tumor had to be removed, even if it took some extraordinary measures on the part of the operating team.

Draining her spinal column appeared to lower the pressure enough to proceed.

Larry told us how he was then able to remove a circular section of skull about the size of the circle you can make if you hold your thumbs and your index finger in the form of the letter C.

Under the skull there is a tough lining that covers the brain and protects it from coming into direct contact with the bony skull. When the section of skull was removed, the brain lining swelled up into the opening. There remained a great deal of pressure inside Michele's tiny head.

As Larry carefully removed that section of lining, the tumor, straining for more room, split an opening in the brain and poked itself up out of Michele's head.

"All I had to do then was to incise that split in her brain into a full incision," he said.

The tumor had crushed a small portion of Michele's brain against the skull. That piece of brain material, about the size of a quarter, was all the brain tissue that had to be removed during the operation.

Larry, working very carefully, then removed the smooth, brown, ugly tumor from Michele's brain. That part of the operation took only a short time. The enemy was placed in a stainless steel bowl. It would be taken to the lab, when the surgery was over, to be thoroughly examined and identified.

All the tiny bleeders in Michele's brain were then either tied off or cauterized, a very time consuming, demanding task.

The brain, Larry explained, does not have the ability to absorb blood, so they can't leave any vein, or even capillary unsealed to leak after they close the skull. They do not want even a single drop of blood released, after they close.

Now that the tumor, which measured about ten centimeters — or about the size of a tennis ball — had been removed, Larry put on a pair of microscopic binoculars. For the next several hours, he meticulously examined the entire tumor bed, cell by cell, looking for any abnormal cells. He didn't dare leave behind even a single active cancer cell. He wouldn't get the chance to come this way again.

Michele, meanwhile, was doing just fine. Her heart was strong, her lungs were working fine and her blood pressure was stable. As far as the rest of her body knew, she was just sleeping deeply. It was a long, good rest for this tough kid.

"I don't think we did any major damage to her," he told us. "But, we really don't know. We're working in the motor hemisphere back there where walking, talking and all the other movements of her body are controlled. And you know, you're working with cobwebs in there. There are no color-coded wires," he said with a grin.

"You mean..." I started to say.

"... that she may not be able to talk? That she may not be able to walk? Yes," he finished for me. "But, we won't know until she wakes up."

"However, whatever we've taken away from her during surgery, we can reteach her," he continued.

"The brain is an amazing organ. At this young age, our brain is able to quite easily adapt to being damaged — even heavily damaged. If I've short circuited, for example, the part of her brain that's responsible for talking, another part of the brain will take over and do that job. If the area of the brain that controls the muscles in her legs has been unwired, another part of her brain will assume that role. It might take a while, but I don't think we've taken anything away from her that can't be completely restored — with therapy.

"Now, please understand, I'm not talking about coming back somewhat, like sometimes happens when a person suffers a stroke. I'm talking about all the way back. That's just one of the advantages of being so young. Up to now, so little of her brain has been used."

Larry words were very encouraging to us at that moment.

"I'm also very sure that we got every bit of the tumor out of there. I spent a lot of time looking for individual cells."

Patsy and I both felt like a huge weight had just been lifted off of our backs. We knew she wasn't out of the woods yet. Complete recovery would be a long haul, but she was still alive and apparently none the worst for having had people walking around in her brain all day.

Remembering that we wanted to see her in the recovery room, he said, "Come on, let's go see if she's awake, yet."

Larry was still very high from his tremendous — never before — accomplished medical achievement. He was almost walking on air.

When we entered the recovery room, there she was, laying motionless on a bed along the far side of the room. He head wrapped in a huge white bandage.

"Well," said the recovery room nurse, "She's been telling me that her mom and dad were coming to see her, but I told her that parents didn't usually come in to recovery."

"You mean, she's talking?," Patsy asked.

"Yes. She's only been awake for a few minutes, but she seems to be just fine."

Michele was laying very still, with her eyes closed. She did not appear to be in any pain. Her face had a tired, but very peaceful, look on it.

"Hi, Baby. I love you," I said, kneeling on the floor by the bed.

"I love you too, but I have to go to the bathroom, very badly, Daddy," she said, very, very softly.

My heart skipped the next few beats. She was alive. She was talking. She was just fine!

"Go ahead and go, Honey," Patsy said.

"I'll get the bed wet, Mommy," she reminded Pats.

We all looked at Larry who was just standing there, shaking his head. I wanted to cheer and scream, "Wet the damn bed, who the hell cares?"

"It's okay, Baby. Doctor Grayhair put a tube there so you don't have to get up to go to the bathroom," Patsy said to Michele through her tears of joy.

Michele was completely silent for a few seconds. I thought maybe she had suddenly slipped back over to the other side. I didn't know what to expect next. None of us did. I looked at Larry. Patsy looked at the nurse.

Then Michele said, "Well, I went. But it still feels like I have to go."

We all smiled and grinned and cheered — inside.

"That's just the tube that makes you feel that way. Don't worry about it, just rest," Patsy said.

"How are you feeling?" Larry asked.

"Fine, thank you."

"Are you a little tired?" I asked.

"Yes. I think I'll take a little nap now."

She still hadn't moved a muscle.

"Okay. You get some rest. Mom and I will be back in a little while," I told her as I gently touched her hand.

"Okay," she said, very softy.

We both kissed her and looked down at this tiny baby with the huge, white bandage covering her whole head. She looked so fragile, so vulnerable, but so damn good to us.

We thanked the nurse, asking her to keep a special eye on our prize, then quietly walked out into the hallway with Larry.

"Boy, I'll tell you. That really looks good to me. I'd be surprised if there was any long term damage there at all. She's really an amazing child," Larry said.

"You're the one who's amazing. Thank you, very much," I said, putting my hand on Larry's shoulder.

Then I kissed Patsy.

"I've got to call Charlie. It's been a long day for her, too. I'll meet you back in Michele's room, Pats." I left the two of them standing there in the hall outside the recovery room.

"Are you going to call my mom and dad, as well?," she asked.

"Sure. I'll tell them you'll call tonight, after we get home."

"Thanks, Honey." She gave me that special smile. The one I fell in love with almost eleven years before.

I went down to the lobby. I wanted to sing. I wanted to shout. I wanted to dance. All the energy that had built up during this long, tense day, wanted out. I didn't know what to do. I wanted to scream, kiss people, dance, jump, run; so I did, but not as much as I wanted to.

I'd always thought that Michele was one of a kind, now I knew she really was. It was a wonderful day. I must have had a smile on my face that was a mile wide.

"Hello," said a small voice on the first ring.

"Charlie?"

"Dad! Is Michele okay?"

"She's just great, Baby. Mom and I just left her in recovery. She came through the surgery just fine. There's nothing for you to worry about, Honey. Your little sister is just doing great."

"Patrick's sure going to be glad to hear that, Pop."

Standing there on the phone in the lobby of Childrens Hospital in Boston, telling my oldest daughter the good news about her sister, suddenly the tears just started to flow down my cheeks for the first time that day.

"I know, Baby. I know. I can't wait to tell him."

"What's bald, only three feet tall and glows in the dark?"
"Michele Nolan, of course!"

"Turn off the lights, Michele."
"I already did, Teresa."
"Then pull the blankets over your head so I can get to sleep."

... black comedy seems to enable a person to deal with a problem that might,
without a sense of humor, become too heavy to carry.

Chapter Ten

"You Said It Would Grow Back, Daddy!"

Michele was out of recovery and back up to her room within an hour.
But, once there, she wasn't in any mood to talk or to be entertained. She
just wanted to sleep.

At about six-thirty that evening, we decided that we should say good
night to Michele, leave her in the capable hands of the nursing staff and
that I should head for Sudbury and a good night's sleep. It had been a very
long day.

Patrick elected to return in Boston to keep an important dinner
appointment he had made weeks before with several of the executives
from the television station.

Just as we were leaving, Larry Page made one of his unscheduled visits
to the fourth floor. He just wanted to convince himself that she was really
still with us, I think.

"We did something very special today," he reminded us. "I'm still on
cloud nine."

Larry Page and his surgical team had indeed done something very
special this day. Four months before, Bob Filler and his team had indeed
done something very special. And, of course, Michele Kathleen Nolan had
done something very special. But we hadn't done anything special. Patrick
and I had just picked the weapons.

As Patrick drove me home to Sudbury, before returning to Boston, we
talked about the people we had met during our short time in New England.

There were the Reeds, a young couple with two children who lived
across the street. David was a super salesman, who was buying into the
printing specialties company he worked for, and who would eventually
become one of the country's most successful marketing specialists.

His wife, Carol, was a striking blond who had an amazing feel for
what looked good in her home, in her clothes and on her children. Carol
was able to discover some of the best bargains in furniture, accents and
just plain "stuff" around New England, and add them to a room so that
the room had just the right feel to it. She had a real talent which she
probably could have sold, but she devoted most of her time to the care of

her children and her husband, David.

There are days when I miss the Reeds. I hope they think kindly of us, from time to time. We do of them.

Then there was that wonderful man, George DeGrasse, the president of a local bank, who lived just across the way from us. George had been an amateur entertainer in college. He could still play the piano and sing a little when we met him. By then, he was in his sixties. George loved to invite people over the the house, put on a bright red sports jacket, sit down at the piano and bang out a tune or two.

George's wife, Alma, was a delightfully warm woman. She kept a common blue jay in the screened porch for two years after rescuing it with a broken wing and nursing it back to health. She couldn't bare to let it fly free for fear that it was so used to being cared for that it wouldn't survive on its own in the wild.

George always indulged Alma's wishes, no matter how bizarre. I don't think they ever did get all the bird droppings out of that screen porch, after the bird died of old age.

One day, I was telling George, who was originally from Maine, how both Patrick and I had been so surprised at the warm welcome we had received when we moved to Massachusetts.

"George," I said, "I was always told that the native New Englander was cold and distant, particularly to strangers and people who were native to another part of the country."

"Patsy, we're just as friendly and warm as most folks. A course," he said, raising one eyebrow, "we do like our privacy."

He made that wonderful comment, slightly exaggerating his clipped, downeast accent.

We've laughed at that story for years. George and Alma DeGrasse were wonderful people and wonderful neighbors.

Directly across the street from us lived a couple of school teachers and their two kids. Lynn Adams and her first husband are divorced now, but during the first few months we lived there, they were very good neighbors. Such good neighbors, in fact, that one day, during that week before Michele's brain surgery and a few days before Patrick's Mom arrived, Lynn and her mom, "Nani," broke into our house.

We had been coming home from the hospital at around ten each night, fixing a quick snack for dinner, throwing the dishes in the sink, dropping our clothes in the hamper (or on the floor in the bedroom), falling into bed for a few hours of fitful sleep, getting up before dawn and returning to Boston — Patrick to BZ, me to the hospital for the day.

The night before the surgery, we came home particularly late. We'd stayed with Michele until nine or so and then had stopped for a bite to eat on the way home, knowing that neither of us would feel like even heating up a cup of soup when we got back to Sudbury.

When I walked in the door I thought I was in the wrong house. The dishes were done, the clothes were washed, ironed, folded and put away. The floors were vacuumed, the furniture was dusted and the trash was gone. We'd been invaded by Good Housekeeping.

I couldn't believe my eyes. I had so dreaded having to eventually face that mess, but the mess had disappeared. Who could have done this?

There wasn't much time for an investigation tonight. We went to bed. We'd look into this matter more closely sometime after tomorrow's surgery.

As we drove home from the hospital that night, after the successful surgery, I still didn't know who had been responsible for cleaning our house.

Patrick turned into the driveway. The lights were on in our house. That morning, when we left for Childrens, I had made sure the lights were all out.

"Looks like the elves have returned," Patrick said.

I went into the house, Patrick went down to talk to the Reeds and bring Teresa home.

Within minutes of our arrival, George called. I think he'd been watching for the car.

"Patsy, we're going to order out Chinese, can we get you and Patrick something?," asked sweet George.

I told him that Teresa and I would be eating alone, that Patrick was going to dinner with people at BZ.

"Then I'll get enough for just the two of you," he said and hung up.

Fifteen minutes later, after Patrick had returned with Teresa and left for Boston, George and Alma were at the front door with a large box. In the box were two complete Chinese dinners, which they'd somehow managed to keep hot, and a bottle of bourbon and a bottle of ginger ale. George explained that the dinner was Alma's idea and the bourbon was his. George opened the bottle and poured three drinks.

I thanked both of them for their kindness and their thoughtfulness and for the drink.

"Thanks," I said, lifting the glass to a successful day, "I really needed a little belt tonight, George."

"I figured you might, but I also figured that you wouldn't want to drink alone."

Since that day I've often smiled — and cried — about that wonderful, neighborly, friendly and intuitive gesture of George and Alma's.

The DeGrasses told me that Carol Reed was the one who had passed the word of Michele's successful surgery through the neighborhood. George and Alma told her that they'd handle our dinner. After a little persuading — and another drink or two, George finally told me who had invaded our house the day before with mops, brooms and dust cloths.

It turned out that Lynn Adams and her mom, whom everyone — children, grandchildren, friends, neighbors, everyone — called, Nani, had been the invading housekeepers — the elves. Nani was a round, sweet lady of Italian decent.

For Nani, cleaning our house while we were in the middle of a crisis was just the neighborly thing to do. Besides, Nani couldn't stand a dirty house. Our house had never before been asked to endure such a thorough cleaning. I think she even dusted the molding above all the windows.

I'll never be able to properly thank all the wonderful people who lived in our neighborhood on Old Meadow Road and the surrounding streets, nor all the others from Sudbury, Brookline, Boston and Lexington who were so warm, thoughtful and kind during those difficult and stressful days.

We never could have gotten through those days without the kind, loving folks who gave us their hearts, their good thoughts, their strong support and their dust cloths.

The night after Michele's brain surgery, Patrick and I took Bob Filler and his wife, June out to dinner. We wanted to thank them for being good friends, as well as for being our baby's caring physician.

Patrick selected a restaurant in the very Italian North End of Boston, which was owned and operated by a wildly eccentric lady, known the world over as simply, Felicia. I don't think I ever heard Felicia's last name, but I think it must have been very Italian. Patrick had somehow discovered Felicia and had asked her to be a semi-regular guest chef on the morning show. She quickly developed into a full blown Boston celebrity.

Felicia was a great guest on the morning show. She has this wonderful, slightly Italian accented, deep, throaty voice. It's not a soft, warm — Gina Lollobrigida — type voice. It's more like the sound one makes when you're walking on a pebbled path while wearing golf shoes. She also always seems to be just slightly out of breath, whenever you meet her.

Filled with enthusiasm for great food, Felicia is a real, wonderful, Boston character. Patrick often used Felicia to soften the show between the appearances of people with a cause, a book to sell or a politician leaders, like his friend, Michael Dukakis, who was in those days a young legislator from Brookline with his eye on the Governor's office.

One of the Boston Globe reporters , who used to catch the show regularly, watched one morning when Felicia was on cooking a "Roman Meal" over a glowing barbecue. She had a whole twelve pound sea bass on the coals. There she was, in a cocktail dress and high heels at nine-thirty in the morning, cooking fish over a bed of hot coals on television.

Three weeks later there was a major — cover story — feature article, complete with pictures, on the front page of the Living Section of the Sunday Globe. Felicia was no longer a local TV guest, she was a star.

Sooner or later, everybody who was anybody — or thought they were — could be seen climbing the steep, narrow stairs to Felicia's place on the second floor in Boston's Italian North End.

Felicia's place soon became known as THE place to go in Boston. Felicia's place was also rumored to be the favorite restaurant of some of the Boston mafia, as well. There was one room there which was often curtained off from the main dining room. I'm sure those were the times when one of the Dons was dining there with his "associates."

Boston's North End was, and still is, like the Vatican in Rome, a city within a city. It's a wonderful part of the city to visit, but, unless your name ends in a vowel, don't plan to live there.

Felicia's restaurant, which was upstairs, over an Italian bakery, on a narrow, hard to find, side street, became one of the most popular restaurants in Boston. People came from all over to eat at Felicia's, and to meet the cook.

In later years, Bob Hope flew her out to California to supervise the meals at his big golf tournament in Palm Desert. Everyone who is anyone eats at least one meal at Felicia's when they visit to Boston.

You can't go to Felicia's without being captivated by this outrageous, ageless lady. On most nights in those days, Felicia did all the cooking.

Several times each evening, between preparing steaming plates of green fettucini, veal marsala and eggplant parmesan, Felicia would sweep out of the kitchen, dressed in a lovely cocktail dress and high heels, to greet her favorite guests. It was always a great treat to have Felicia spend a few minutes standing at your table or the table of a special guest, a regular or celebrity. The walls are plastered with photos of Felicia and hundreds of, as she calls them, "Just a few of my friends."

Her sons and a nephew run the dining room, doubling as greeters, waiters and jacks-of-all-trades, but Felicia ran the kitchen. She cooked everything to order.

Felicia is just one of the wonderful characters I met while Patrick was producing television shows.

On this particular evening at Felicia's, not only was her favorite television producer — the guy who helped make her into a Boston celebrity — there with his lady for dinner, but he'd brought along a world famous pediatric surgeon, Dr. Robert Filler and his wife, June. It was an unbelievable night of dining and wining, punctuated by periodic visits from the cook. Felicia exploded from the kitchen the minute Anthony told her Patrick was there. Hugs and kisses for everyone.

"Patrick," she growled in her whiskey voice, "Let me cook for you and your friends tonight, please."

We were not allowed to even glance at a menu. Felicia was in her glory.

The night would begin with a bottle of champagne — after all, didn't we have to toast the world renowned surgeon and his lady? Then the whole room had to toast the new celebrity — more champagne.

Next came little appetizers, then chicken, followed by veal, followed by a delicate pasta in a delicious oyster sauce, followed by more food from Felicia's boundless kitchen.

Each new course, of course, included another bottle of fine Italian wine. Finally, when no one could move, she had a huge plate of cannoli (a delicious Italian dessert) sent to the table. It was a night to remember. We were lucky to survive.

The night included a call by the world famous surgeon to Michele's nurse at Childrens Hospital. Bob just wanted to be sure everything was still okay. It was. Michele was sleeping peacefully. Back to the feast.

We could barely walk down the stairs to the street after three hours of Felicia's Italian cooking. We were, of course, also carrying two huge baskets filled to the brim with cheese, salami, desserts and wine.

We never left Felicia's without... " a little something to take home to the children."

The children never saw a bite of what we had in those baskets.

After dinner with Felicia, Bob wanted to see where Patrick worked. It seems that he was as fascinated with Patrick's broadcasting world as Patrick has always been was with Bob's world of medicine.

So, feeling little pain, after the wine and the champagne and the meal, which had been forced on us by our hostess, we paid a late night visit to the studios of WBZ-TV and WBZ radio.

There is, (or at least was in those days) on late night BZ radio, an unusual — some say completely bizarre — talk show host. His name is

Larry Glick (really, his name is Glick). Larry doesn't do politics and he doesn't do controversy — but he does do weird. He does weird with a wacky, wonderful, offbeat sense of humor.

With a station pumping out 50,000 watts of clear channel power, Larry finds a lot of company out there after dark. As we were touring BZ, we naturally stopped in to pay a call on "The Glickster."

Glick immediately wanted to know who we had brought into his world from the real world. In seconds the prominent pediatric surgeon, Dr. Robert Filler, M.D., was on the air, talking about Michele, pediatric medicine and life in general to the thirty-two states and five foreign countries which are reached by WBZ radio at night. Bob loved every minute of it.

Two days later, and for weeks after that, boxes started arriving at Childrens Hospital with bears, dolls and toys. Michele got thousands and thousands of get well cards and notes from all over the eastern part of the United States and Canada. The mail came by the sackful — too many letters and cards to ever answer personally.

A few days later, I went back on Glick's show to thank everyone who had written — and to ask them to please stop sending cards, bears, pandas and dolls. The second appearance precipitated even more cards, dolls and stuffed animals. Michele kept a few of the hundreds of stuffed bears, pandas, lions, tigers, cats, giraffes and children's books which arrived. We gave the rest to children all over the hospital. For some, it was an early visit from Santa.

Several of the people who heard about Michele that night on the Glick show and who took the time to write a personal note, wrote more than once. One lady, from a small town in the Midwest, wrote to Michele regularly for over five years. Patsy, with a little help from Michele, answered all of her letters. One day we got a note from the woman's daughter. Michele's pen pal had died, peacefully, in her sleep (listening to the madness of The Glickster, I presume). The daughter just wanted to thank Michele for reaching out to her house-bound mom.

Within a day or two of the surgery Michele was up and about, feeling stronger each day. Since the surgery had been to her head, she didn't have to recover from the same painful invasion of her abdomen as she had suffered on the first two surgeries. The post operative recovery from brain surgery is almost painless since no muscles or nerves have been cut or damaged. Her head was still wrapped in an enormous white bandage and she wasn't really happy about her appearance. She didn't like the look of that big dressing. Each day she would fuss to someone about that big white dressing on her head. She wanted it removed, but, of course, it had to stay.

One day, Charlie Austin arrived with a picture of himself. The picture had been taken a couple of years before, when Charlie had undergone emergency brain surgery to correct an aneurysm.

There, in the picture, was our friend Charlie, with his head enclosed in a bandag identical to the one on Michele's head. After that, the dressing wasn't an issue with Michele. If it was good enough for Charlie Austin, it was good enough for her. There wasn't another word about it.

170

A few days after the surgery, Larry asked if he could talk to me, for a moment, privately. We went into a small conference room near the nurse's desk.

"The Head Nurse has requested that since Michele is no longer critical, you now observe the same visiting hours as everyone else. Would that be a problem for you?"

I couldn't believe it. For the past four days, when Michele didn't need my attention, I had bathed the other children in the ward and changed their beds. When things on the floor got busy or hectic with a problem, I had taken every available patient — some of them in wheelchairs, others in carts and others walking, out onto the screen porch and read a story to them. Every afternoon I read to all who wished to gather on the porch. I was saving that nurse dozens of staff hours, I had read scores of books to the kids — including "The Grinch" about fifty times — and now, for some unspoken reason, I was no longer welcome here, except during regular visiting hours — 2 to 4 in the afternoon and 6 to 8 in the evening.

I carefully explained to Larry the things I had been doing, not just for our daughter, but for all the patients on the fourth floor. I was really upset. Hadn't she been paying any attention?

"What she doesn't understand is that I've been where she is. I've done her job. But she hasn't been where I am. She hasn't done my job. She just doesn't understand that the most important thing up here is Michele. The second most important person is you and she's a poor third. I'm really upset with her attitude. It isn't like I was in the way or asking her to get me a cup of coffee. I've been making a real contribution to this place, every day."

Larry listened to me and then asked, "What time do you usually get here in the morning, Patsy?"

"I'm usually here a little after seven. I ride in with Patrick."

"And what time do you leave in the evening?"

"We're always out of here by the end of visiting hours, eight o'clock."

"Sounds fine to me."

He walked out of the conference room and went to the nurses station.

"May I have Michele Nolan's chart, please."

He opened the chart to the order sheet and wrote: "Mrs. Nolan may visit Michele between the hours of 6am and 9pm, without restriction." Then he signed the order.

"That should cover it," he said.

The sad part of this story is that from then on, the Head Nurse treated me as though I were a VIP. She offered to get me coffee, told me that there were donuts in the lounge and offered to get me a better chair. That really pissed me off.

Why wasn't I special when I was helping her and the other nurses with the work load — which I kept right on doing, of course — and not just when I gained some kind of special guest status when a doctor wrote an order?

In another day or two, things calmed down and we returned to our normal routines. I bathed the kids, changed the beds and read to whoever needed attention and she stopped asking me if I wanted a donut.

Larry Page wanted Michele to stay in the hospital for a full ten days. It was critical that the brain not spring a leak. She couldn't survive even a slight seepage from one of the many blood vessels that had been cut. If one of them did begin to bleed, she'd have to return to surgery to have it repaired, immediately.

So, for ten days, feeling relatively well for at least eight of those days, Michele remained confined to the fourth floor at Childrens. She wasn't living on the eighth floor, the oncology floor, where all the children were suffering from some form of cancer, she was on a surgical floor. She spent most of her day visiting the other kids on the floor. She walked around wearing a new, pink bathrobe that went all the way to the floor. The hem cleared the floor by about a half an inch. It was so funny to watch her as she walked about the hospital. Since the bathrobe flared out quite a bit at the bottom, you never saw her legs. You couldn't even see them move under the robe. It looked like a wind up doll was moving from room to room on wheels.

One day Patrick noticed that Michele seemed to be doing a lot of yawning. He asked Larry if there was something wrong. Had her blood chemistry become unbalanced or something, Patrick asked.

"She's just bored," Larry said.

"Pardon me?"

"She's bored. She's talked to every patient, had every book in the library read to her — including the Doctor Seuss book, "How the Grinch Stole Christmas at least five hundred times — she's talked to every gray lady and played with every toy. She's just bored, but she knows she can't go home until Tuesday, so she yawns. It'll stop when she goes home," Larry said casually.

It was just another convincing piece of evidence, even at four, that she was the most pragmatic person anyone has ever known. If fussing about something wasn't going to change anything — and fussing to go home was, after all, known to her to be a lost cause — then why bother to fuss?

She's like that today. If discussing it might change the situation, she can become a powerful advocate. But if she sees that a protest is futile, she just accepts the inevitable. As a result, she lives a much more peaceful life than most of us. It's truly a wonderful gift.

That Doctor Seuss book, the one about the Grinch stealing Christmas, was so thoroughly memorized during all those readings, that now, more than twenty years later, it remains an important part of each Christmas eve's activities. This past year she was pleased to recite the entire book, completely from memory, to her two year old niece, Alicia.

Michele even has a big Grinch doll that accompanies the story. "... and the Grinch, himself, carved the roast beast."

For every one of the millions of parents who have read a Dr. Seuss book to a sick child, we would like to say, Thank you, Dr. Seuss. You too helped in Michele's recovery.

Within a few days I developed a light fuzz under the bandage. But then, the radiation treatments to the tumor bed — just in case Larry had missed a cell or two in there — began. The radiation treatments continued every day for six weeks.

Just as I was developing a semblance of a crew cut hairdo after the surgery (Dad took one really nice picture of me during that time. It's the one on page 15, just before Chapter One), the effects of the radiation took over and all my hair fell out. I was now completely and totally, bald.

There wasn't a trace of fuzz anywhere on my entire head. That may seem like a traumatic experience for a little kid, but at four, that condition is only a minor inconvenience. In fact, it can actually become the basis for some rather bizarre horseplay, especially if you have a sense of humor that sometimes tends to be on the dark side, like I do.

Now, I don't know if I was born with that dark sense of humor or whether it developed as a result of being close to death at a young age. But I do know that all the kids who I knew who had cancer, and my own family, tended to make dark jokes about having cancer. It was, as Dad says, kind of a junior version of gallows humor.

"What's bald, only three feet tall and glows in the dark?"
"Michele, of course."
"Turn off the lights, Michele."
"I did."
"Then pull the blankets over your head so I can get to sleep."

I guess the black comedy enables a person to deal with a problem that might, without a sense of humor about it, become too heavy to bare.

I had received, from a variety of sources, several interesting caps, hats and head covers. Most of the time I was happy to be bareheaded in the house, but as the winter grew cool, I'd wear one of my silly or funny hats when we went out.

Dad bought me a wig. It was an inexpensive, stretch wig that Mom altered to fit my tiny head. It had gobs of black curls. I didn't have fuzz.

One of my favorite tricks was to wear the wig out in public — I particularly liked to wear the wig when the family went out to dinner. I would sit there quietly, a small, almost gaunt child, wearing a thick head of synthetic hair. The waiter would come to take our order, which should normally only take a few minutes to give. But, I always insisted on placing my own order, even if I was having the same thing as all the others at the table. I wanted to make sure the waiter paid particular attention to me because as soon as the waiter left the table, I would hide the wig under the table, on my lap.

Then, when he returned with his arms loaded with plates of food, the waiter would discover that one of the children he was about to serve was now completely, stark raving bald. I used to shock a lot of folks in those days. It was a great game.

One day, Mom and my brother Patrick and I were at the Faneuil Hall Market Place in Boston. Patrick was in a stroller and I was watching him for Mom as she shopped. This particular day I had pulled off my hat — it was warm in the market — and stashed it in the stroller with the diaper bag and my coat. I never wore the wig if I had one of my crazy caps or hats on my head. Together, they were just too much.

So, there I was completely bald, wearing pants. My brother, Patrick, on the other hand, had long, blond curls and was bundled up in the stroller.

"Oh, little boy, I see you're helping your mother take care of your little sister," said a well meaning lady who was also shopping in the market.

173

"He's my brother and I'm a girl. I'm a girl with no hair, but I'm a girl," I said firmly.

The lady just covered her mouth and walked on. She had been wrong on both counts. Mom, who was standing nearby, loved it. Boy indeed, I thought.

Lots of people would mistake me for a boy in those days when I was completely bald. I think even more people actually thought I was a boy when the hair eventually started to grow back. Girls just didn't have crew cuts in those days, though some do, today.

Dad says that no matter how delicate or feminine or ladylike a little girl is, even dressed in a pretty pink dress, if they're bald, they still look like a little boy. It's a social expectation, Dad says. Boys have short hair, girls have long hair. For nine months when I was four and five years old, I had no hair at all.

Three weeks after the surgery, Michele was gaining strength and feeling good. The rest of the family all came down with a raging case of the flu. Michele seemed to be fine.

The next night, as I was tucking in the kids, I noticed that Michele was acting very strangely. She didn't seem to be able to control her eyes.

No matter where she looked, her eyes looked to the side, even when they should have looked straight ahead.

It's a little hard to describe, exactly, but she seemed to be visually disoriented, but didn't seem to be able to recognize it. I got a little scared.

"Patrick, can you come here and take a look at Michele, please."

We put Michele in our bed. She even walked sideways.

"Honey, can you see me?," Patrick asked.

"Yes," came the answer as her eyes looked toward the far wall and not toward Patrick at all.

"Where am I?"

"Right there," she said, a little impatiently, as she correctly pointed toward him, as her eyes looked to the left — almost as if she was looking around a corner. Suddenly, it became very scary.

She didn't seem to be able to look at anything you asked her to look at. She was confused and starting to get a little scared herself.

"Daddy, what's wrong?," she said through her tears.

"Honey, I don't know," was all Patrick could offer.

"Let's call Larry."

I called Larry's house. The baby sitter said he was out for the evening. He was playing poker at a friend's house, she said, but she had the number, which she gave me.

I got Larry Page on the phone in just a minute or two. When I told him of Michele's symptoms, he asked me three questions.

"Does she complain of a headache?"

"No."

"Does she have a fever?"

"No."

"Have any of the kids had the flu recently?"

"They all have it now. All but Michele."

"Nothing to worry about. It's just the flu," he said as his voice relaxed.

He explained that when Michele contracted the flu it didn't behave like it would in a normal child. The flu virus had attacked the weakest part of Michele's body, the freshly wounded place in her brain where the tumor had been removed. The swelling — which hadn't caused any discomfort because there was now room for her brain to expand into the void left behind when the tumor was removed — was responsible for her strange, and frightening, disorientation.

Larry said he would call our druggist and have a prescription delivered. The drug would relieve the situation.

"It's a drug which we normally prescribe — almost routinely — as a post operative prophylactic, but she seemed to tolerate the surgery so well that I didn't think it was necessary. I'll call your drug store. Give her two pills tonight and then one a day starting in the morning," Larry said.

"How long should she take it," I asked.

"Oh, probably for the next two years," he said calmly.

Within twenty minutes, our wonderful drug store, Post Road Apothecary, in Sudbury, delivered a small bottle of tablets. I gave Michele two pills and put her to bed. She went right to sleep.

I don't think Patrick and I slept for more than two or three hours that night. We just lay there, holding hands, worrying about what was happening inside that tiny head in the next room. We'd drop off the sleep, but wake up, worried about Michele.

The next day was Saturday, so Patrick didn't have to get up before dawn and go to the studio. We both were awake when the sun came up.

"I don't want to go see how she is. I'm scared she might not be there," Patrick said.

"I know. I feel the same way. I'm terrified of what I might find when I walk into her room."

We both just lay there, staring at the ceiling. We were scared silly, all over again.

In a few minutes, the door to our bedroom burst open and through it walked a bright, happy, completely normal Michele Kathleen.

"Good morning," she said.

"Are you okay, this morning?"

"Yes. I'm fine. Are we ever going to get some breakfast around here?"

Patrick and I laughed and then cried, pulling Michele up onto the bed with us. Her eyes were back to normal. The disorientation was completely gone. It was the most amazing thing I have ever seen.

We had a really wonderful Saturday breakfast that day.

For the next two years we started each morning with a glass of juice and a pill. There was just that one instance of disorientation. It was a terrible night that neither Patrick nor I will ever forget, but there was just that incident. After two years, we discontinued the medication.

The day before Christmas that year I was suddenly confronted by a completely bald, twenty-seven pound prosecutor.

"Dad, didn't you say my hair would grow back?," she demanded.

"Yes, Honey, it will. It's just that about the time it started to grow back all the radiation made it fall out. Doctor Grayhair tells me that it will grow back eventually, but it may take a while. Why are you suddenly so troubled by being bald? You keep playing those mean jokes on people with

175

that wig of yours."

"Cause everybody else has a Christmas bow in their hair and I don't have any hair for a bow," she said — with a semi-pout on her face. She was pretending to be vary indignant, but was, as usual, pulling hard on her daddy's willing leg.

"I can fix that, Beulah Baldy! I can fix anything," I assured her.

I went into the den, where all the Christmas wrappings were kept, and returned with a bright red, stick-on bow. I pealed the paper backing from the adhesive and stuck the bow right on Michele's bald head, just to the side, exactly where a bow might be placed if Patsy had actually tied one in her hair for Christmas.

Michele was very pleased. I took a picture of her in her blue satin Christmas dress, with the white lace collar, and the bright red bow on her head. The next day, she wore another red bow all day, clear through Christmas dinner.

As the credo she would later adopt as her own says, "If the world doesn't fit, make adjustments."

About nine months after her surgery, Michele's hair came out of its dormant stage and started slowly — very slowly — to grow. Her hair returned as very fine baby hair. The area where the tumor had been, the back left quarter of her head, had received much more radiation than had the rest of her head, so that circular portion of her scalp remains without any hair to this day.

As it is, her hair only grows about an inch each year on the rest of her head. It took a long time before she looked like a girl. It was even longer before her first post operative haircut.

During those bald days, Michele was, of course, branded with a series of nicknames, by her loving family. Beulah Baldy was only one. Harriet Hairyhead was my favorite. The name Priscilla Petalpuss was reserved for those days when she choose to wear her big, floppy hat with pink flaps all over it. She actually liked that silly hat better than she did the wig.

One day, when she had grown back about three inches of hair, she decided that the wig had outlived it's usefulness; at least it had for her. She packed the wig in with her other stuff when we went to Boston for her next chemotherapy visit and gave it to the doctors at the Jimmy Fund.

"Some other little girl can use this now. I don't need it anymore," she told Dr. Traggis.

In addition to the radiation, the doctors at the Jimmy Fund elected — and we agreed — to a two year course of continued chemotherapy. They chose the drug Actinomycin-D, a powerful, proven cancer fighter in the battle with Wilm's.

The drug was a terrible shock to Michele's whole system. It took away her appetite, it caused her to just feel lousy all over, and it just kind of "stopped" her.

It was after all, as they explained, poisoning all her cells. The normal cells would be able to endure the poison — with some stress — but the cancer cells died from the poison. She got a shot of Actinomycin-D every day for seven days in a row, then nothing for a month. After three weeks, just as she was feeling almost back to normal, it was time to start the next course of treatment.

Before each shot she had to submit to a blood test. Normally, the lab technician would take one small, bony finger, jab a sharp stylist into it and extract a small amount of blood for the test. As there were seven shots in a week, there were seven blood tests in a week.

Michele soon found out that if they hit the same finger two days in a row it was twice as painful, so she, in her typically pragmatic way, made a deal with the ladies of the lab. She knew they had to do the test, that she did not fuss about. Fussing wasn't, after all, going to cancel the test, just delay it and give everyone a little extra aggravation, which they did not need. So she didn't fuss about having the test, she just didn't like the methods they used, so she made a deal.

Her deal was, if she got to choose which finger got jabbed, she wouldn't cry — at all. She wouldn't, she said, even cry out. As that horrible blade struck a tiny digit, she would simply utter the word, "Oh."

Just a very quiet, "Oh," and nothing more, was all she would say.

It was a good deal for everybody, but I don't know how she kept from crying out when that cold, steel blade sliced into her tiny finger.

My favorite lab technician was a large — and I mean large — lady named Pearl. Pearl called me, the Mushroom Girl. She said that I was so little that she thought I probably lived under a mushroom somewhere in the woods of Sudbury.

All of the people at the Jimmy Fund were great with kids. They had to be; that's all they ever saw. They had games and stories and a way of making it easier on the kids, without actually lying to any of us.

The walls were all decorated with huge cartoon characters. There were lots of little chairs and little tables in every area. There were books and games and toys. It was a pretty cheerful place when you consider that the only thing they did there, day in and day out, was treat children who were in danger of dying from cancer.

Through all the tests and the drugs and the x-ray treatments, I don't think I ever seriously considered the prospect that I might actually die. Of course, at four, dying is a rather strange concept to grasp. I knew what dying was when it came to animals, but I never remember anyone I knew — when I was that young — dying. I knew dying was not a good thing to happen, so therefore I knew it wouldn't happen to me.

When a treatment would be scheduled on Saturday, to spell Patsy, I usually made the trip to the Jimmy Fund with Michele. After all the trips Patsy had made, even when she was pregnant, it was the very least I could do in return.

One Saturday, after a year or so of seven days on — thirty days off, Michele and I left for Boston right after breakfast.

"Let's get this over with, Kiddo," I said as the Mustang pulled out onto Horse Pond Road.

By now, Michele had the routine down cold. She didn't want me in the lab for the blood test — that part she always did, alone.

She did, however, want me to hold her hand while the doctor injected the drug through a vein in the back of her hand during the treatment. She also didn't want to have the band aid applied to the spot where the needle had been stuck into her. She would take the band aid with her, and in the car, or later at home if she had forgotten to bring one, she stuck that band aid on one of her dolls. All the dolls in the house were, at one time or another, treated for cancer by Michele.

After her treatment, she would hold a small piece of cotton on the tiny wound for fifteen minutes rather than have that band aid applied to her hand.

On this particular day, as we got back into the car, she removed the cotton. The wound had not quite closed so a small bubble of blood appeared on the back of her hand where the needle had been inserted into the vein.

"Michele, let me have that band aid. I don't want any of that drug to leak out of your vein and get under the skin," I said calmly.

Calm was not what I got in return.

"DRUG?"

She spun around in her seat, got up on her knees and stuck her face right into mine.

"You let them put a drug in me?," she hollered in all seriousness.

"Dad, don't you know that drugs are bad?" This little bald tyke was getting very indignant with me.

"Give me the band aid and we'll talk about it," I said.

After I saw that the bleeding was not going to continue, a twenty minute discussion about drugs took place there in the car at the side of The Jimmy Fund. This little kid was very serious about drugs and what was an appropriate use of them when it came to her own body.

We talked about good drugs, bad drugs and good drugs that are used badly by some people. Bad drugs that are against the law. Good drugs that are used by bad people. Drugs like aspirin. Drugs like pain pills. Drugs like the one they had just injected into her hand.

While I may have given a great talk about drugs, it didn't matter much. Television won. Michele had heard that you didn't take drugs, period. But now I had let them put a drug in her. What's wrong with this picture?

It wasn't until we got home, and she confronted her mother — who had by now, suddenly and conveniently, returned to being a nurse as well as being just a mommy — that she let up on me. It was just one of the those things we had not dealt with before it happened.

Finally, only partly convinced by her in-house medical authority that the drug she had received was okay, Michele accepted that maybe — just maybe — I hadn't committed a felony after all. I was paroled, but with certain reservations on the part of the one-child parole board.

I guess Patsy and the doctor had never called it a drug. I do know that I was subjected to an hour of heat from a five year old over my obvious ignorance to the well publicized dangers of drugs.

Needless to say, when Michele became a teenager, illegal drugs held no attraction for her whatsoever. She's still very adamant about the abnormal or illegal use of drugs.

So, be careful what you say to a five year old about drugs, especially if you've just allowed someone to put one into their body. I never referred to it as a "drug" again.

"I' d like you to go right over to Framingham General
and have them give Michele a shot of gamma globulin,
I'll call them and tell them you're coming.
Then I want you to find a place where Michele can stay
while the Chicken Pox runs its course through the family."

Chapter Eleven

Another New Brother & A New Sister!

As the winter passed into spring, I was gaining ground each day, feeling more and more like a normal child. But, then, what did I know about being a normal child?

I'd had two major surgeries when I was three, brain surgery at four and had been receiving monthly doses of a powerful, cancer killing drug for two years. I'd lost all my hair, heard from strangers all over the country, been radiated until I glowed in the dark — or so I used to tease, had been stuck with four thousand needles, had endured liver scans, brain scans, electroencephalograms, EKGs and absorbed what seemed like a million diagnostic x-ray to my kidney, chest, brain and skeleton.

In April of 1970, Dad was offered a great new job. The people of Boston who were trying to improve the conditions at the zoos in Boston asked Dad to bring his promotion and public relations skills and come to work for them. It was a big challenge, but Dad was getting a little tired of getting up at five each morning only to have to deal with guests who thought the end was near, the children had to be saved, the world had to be saved or the country was going to hell in a handbag. After a long talk with Mom, Dad decided to take the job as Public Relations Director for the Boston Zoological Society. Can you imagine how much fun that was going to be for Teresa and me? Our Dad was going to own a zoo.

With all the contacts Dad had with the radio and television stations in New England and at the Boston Globe, he successfully promoted the season's opening of the Children's Zoo. It was the biggest day the zoo had ever had — up to that time.

Teresa got to ride the baby elephant. I wore my wig and got to feed the baby goats and ride on a huge turtle. It was a wonderful spring day in New England and we were all on the television news that night, too. Teresa and I were really going to like this new job of Dad's.

Spring melted into summer and we made frequent trips to the Children's Zoo. Dad was appearing on television regularly, speaking at various service clubs around the Boston area. Mom was busy finding things to amuse her three children. Sometime during that summer, Teresa and I started to get wind of a new "family" plan.

Mom and Dad had always wanted to have a big family, but they also felt that producing more than three children was just plain irresponsible, given the exploding growth in the world's population. Dad calls it, indelicately, People Pollution.

So, one day, they told us that they were thinking about adding a new kid to the family, through adoption. We both thought it was a wonderful idea. The more the merrier, as far as we were concerned.

"Now, you both understand that this new kid, if indeed we do adopt a kid, will be a full fledged member of this family? There will be no, 'you're not really a Nolan,' business. If we adopt a kid, he'll be a Nolan, just like you two and Patrick," Mom told us.

"Sure," we agreed. "Can we pick out the kid we want?," Teresa wanted to know.

"Well, of course you can help," Mom said.

"I want another sister," I said immediately.

"Actually, we were thinking about adopting a little boy to balance things out in the family. Two boys, two girls," said Dad.

"Fine. Patrick needs a brother," said Teresa.

It was just that simple. Add a kid? Fine by us. No big deal.

The next steps went a lot faster than you might imagine.

First, Mom and Dad weren't interested in adopting a baby; they'd had three babies. They also knew that there was probably zero chance of them being given a new baby, what with having three kids already and being perfectly able to produce another child, if they choose to do so. They, instead, talked to an adoption agency that dealt with a group of kids sadly but accurately called, The Unadoptables.

Unadoptables, it seems, are children who are not perfect. Just like many grocery shoppers who only want to buy perfect tomatoes — when they all taste the same — many people only want to adopt a perfect baby. As a result, there are thousands of kids in foster homes waiting, many in vain, for a family they may never get. Some of these kids have physical problems or emotional difficulties. There are also many kids who's only mark against them is that they're not white. Many of the unadoptables are kids who are black, or partly black. It seems that very few black people adopt and very few white people adopt black kids.

So, there we were, faced with accepting a new kid who might be looking at years of medical treatments, months of mental health sessions or at adopting a child who's only sin was being born black — probably to a teenage mother, out of wedlock, Mom told us.

Mom didn't think she could deal with another kid who had to be driven to the hospital all the time and Dad wasn't sure that it was fair to the kids who were already here to bring an unbalanced or disturbed kid into our group.

I'm sure, after seeing how they handled my problems, that they would have dealt just fine with either of those situations, but we'll never know.

Mom and Dad met with the social workers first, to discuss the situation, explaining what they had decided. Teresa, Patrick and I went on the second visit. The social worker was a very gentle lady who showed us a big book, filled with pictures and little descriptions of children who were available for adoption. Teresa and I liked a family of three boys, but Mom got a little pale when we said we wanted all three of them, so we didn't push it.

Before we left the adoption agency we picked out three boys that we wanted to know more about. The social worker said she would call when she had some more information. We went to lunch.

In a week or so we returned to the adoption agency. They had some news. The social worker showed us a couple of recent pictures of a four year old boy — born just five months after me. His name was Michael.

Michael was healthy and seemed to be without any emotional or mental problems. He was shy and didn't talk much, she said, but he had a nice smile.

"Now," said the social worker, "I have a question for you which may surprise you. Would there be any possibility that you might consider adopting two children?"

"Two!," exclaimed Mom. "Why two?"

"Well, Michael has been in the same foster home since he was born. It's a very stable family and they have three or four older children of their own. Michael hasn't been moved around from place to place, like a lot of our kids. Three days after Michael was born a little girl was born and she was also placed in the same foster home, at birth. They have been together since birth and they're both available. Of course, we'll be happy to place Michael with you because we want as many of our children to be adopted as we can find homes for, but we'd sure love it if we didn't have to split up these two. They're not, of course, biological brother and sister, but they've been raised as though they were for four years."

Teresa and I were very excited. A new little sister. Terrific! Mom and Dad would get their second brother and we'd get a sister in the deal. It was a wonderful idea. We were jumping up and down. Patrick, who was only a year old, was sleeping. At his age he couldn't care less about a couple of new kids.

"I don't know if we really want to add two children," Mom said.

"Pats, we've already accepted, in our minds and in the minds of the kids, another child. We're just selecting the one. So, we're not talking about adding two, we're only talking about adding one more," Dad said, trying to place things in proper perspective.

"But, that's five kids," said Mom.

"You were one of seven and it didn't seem to harm you or your brothers and sister," Dad ventured. I think Dad would have adopted ten more kids if he could have talked Mom into it.

"Do you have any information on this little girl?," Mom said, starting to cave in to the pressure, as she nearly always did.

It just so happened that she did have some information. She had a picture of this shy looking, delicate little girl with huge, dark eyes. She looked like she didn't really want to have her picture taken. I still have that wonderful picture of my sister, Traci.

Her name then was Tracy Marie. (Mom and Dad would change the spelling of her first name to Traci when the adoption papers were filed. They also gave Michael a middle name, Sean, when the papers were submitted to the court.)

Traci was bright and, once she got to know you, very outgoing. She did all the talking for both herself and for Michael. It was only one of the reasons Michael didn't talk much. Michael and Traci were living with two teenage foster sisters who, I guess, treated them more like live dolls than a little brother and sister.

I loved the little girl in the photograph immediately. Dad said that maybe what we should do was meet these two children and see what happened. He said it would be better if we met them in a neutral place, informally, so that the two kids didn't feel like they were under any pressure or, in case we didn't adopt them, wouldn't even know they had been rejected. Dad suggested the children's social worker bring them to the Children's Zoo next Saturday.

It was decided that Mom and Dad should meet them first, just to see what the chemistry was like. If that meeting went well, they would make a visit to our home and meet Teresa, Patrick and me. I didn't like the idea of not being included in the first meeting.

"We're all adopting these kids, aren't we?," I wanted to know.

I lost. Mom and Dad went alone to the Children's Zoo.

That first meeting with Mom and Dad went very well. So well, in fact, that the following Wednesday their social worker, a guy named, Ray Chang, brought Michael and Tracy to the house for lunch. Wednesday had been selected because that was only a half school day and Teresa would be home by noon. Dad said he would come home at noon and we could all have lunch together. By the time Dad got there — he's usually late — we had already asked if Tracy and Michael could sleep over. I told you things moved pretty fast.

Finding something for Traci to sleep in that night was hardly a problem since she and I were the same size, but Michael was another matter. He sure couldn't squeeze into anything in Patrick's drawer. Not only did we not have any pajamas for Michael to wear — although we were able to borrow a pair from Mike Adams, across the street — but we didn't have enough beds for everyone.

That first night, Mom and Dad slept in our room in our little beds and Teresa and I and our new little sister, Traci, slept in Mom and Dad's big bed. Michael slept on the extra bed in Patrick's room. Patrick slept in his crib.

In the morning, Ray returned and took Traci and Michael back to their foster home. On Saturday morning, he brought them back for good. By then, Dad had found another bed and Mom had purchased a few boy's things for Michael.

In the space of one short week we had met the new kids and they moved in. We were now seven Nolans. Dad even got a vanity plate for the car with "Nolan 7" on it.

It took two full years before the Commonwealth of Massachusetts made the adoptions of Traci Marie and Michael Sean final. It seems that in those days there were a lot of people who did not approve of interracial adoption — a throwback, I guess, to the old days of miscegenation legislation. Some of the people who still objected included a number of Superior Court Judges. Fran Meaney, a friend of ours, and Dad's lawyer, said that we would have to wait for a sympathetic judge, or at least, one who wouldn't refuse the adoptions on the basis of Michael and Traci being either interracially adopted or without a common religious identification between them and our family. Massachusetts can be a very strange place.

As it turned out, when the mandatory one year waiting period had passed, the folks in the Human Services department at the State House had lost the two applications for adoption. They didn't even have a record of where those two children were living. They had just "lost" two young children.

It took Fran seven months to track down the files — buried under a pile of "dead" files on someone's back desk — and submit the application to the clerk in our county court house — in the famous County of Middlesex. We lived, you see, in the Town of Sudbury, in the County of Middlesex, in The Commonwealth of Massachusetts. I remember the Longfellow poem about The Midnight Ride of Paul Revere, "One if by land and two if by sea, and I on the opposite shore shall be, ready to ride and sound the alarm to every Middlesex Village and farm." We lived in a famous Middlesex village — Sudbury.

After two years of Traci and Michael being Nolans by practice, we entered the huge old Middlesex County Court House one fine fall day to have it all made official. There were the seven Nolans and the four Meaneys. Fran and Pat had invited their two children, Jimmy and Caitlin to witness the proceedings. Everyone was dressed in his best clothes and on his very best behavior. The court house is a scary place, even if you haven't done anything wrong.

We waited and waited and waited. The judge kept us waiting for almost two hours. We had planned to take the Meaneys to lunch after the ceremony, which we thought would take a half an hour, at most. By one-thirty, there were seven real hungry kids, four fairly annoyed parents — who were sick and tired of taking turns holding my brother Patrick — and one very nervous social worker. It was the first time we had seen Ray in over a year and a half.

Finally, the clerk came out ushered us into the judge's chambers. There, behind the desk sat the judge, reading the social worker's report on the family.

When he finished the three page report — while we all tried our best to stand quietly and motionless — he asked, "Which one is Michael?"

Michael raised his hand and looked like he was going to be sent to jail.

"I'll approve this action," he said. "Young man, do you want to make it official?" Michael didn't know what the judge meant. "Here, bang the gavel," said the judge.

Michael picked up the judge's gavel and gave it a fairly sound rap.

"Well, then," said the judge, "That's that." He turned to another matter.

"Excuse me, your honor," said Dad, "but there's a little matter of Traci's adoption."

"Oh, excuse me. I didn't realize these two were related."

With that, he picked up the other social worker report, which, except for the name of the child in question, was identical to Michael's which he had just read with such deliberate care. He made us all stand there, shifting from foot to foot, stomachs' growling, while he carefully read Traci's report. It was so dumb.

"Which one is Traci?," he asked after what seemed to be about three days.

"I am," she said with a clear voice.

"Would you like to make it official?"

Traci didn't have to be asked twice. She grabbed that gavel and smashed it down on the little round block of wood so hard that Dad leapt across the desk and caught the little round block before it bounced into the waste basket. The judge jumped in his seat and Pat Meaney and I just roared with laughter. It was the funniest thing we had seen that day.

Dad said that the whole thing left him feeling a little "shady." It was like something had happened that someone was ashamed of. You see, there were four adults in the room and the judge never once looked at them or even asked which ones were the adoptive parents. He never said, congratulations, good luck, have a nice day or even, goodbye. He hadn't even been concerned enough to notice that there were two kids being adopted. He just signed the papers, let the kids bang the gavel and then he turned to other matters. Dad said it made him real unhappy.

This was supposed to be a wonderful, happy experience — two new children were being added to the family. Instead, we were kept waiting — Dad thinks the judge took a nap — and then the actual adoption was so impersonal and cold. It was good to have had the Meaneys with us. We headed directly across the street to a little restaurant and ordered hamburgers, french fries and "frappes," which is what they call a milk shake in Massachusetts. It turned out to be a happy day — after we got out of that drafty old court house with the inconsiderate judge.

Patsy and I had gotten to know the Meaneys during our second year in Massachusetts. Michael Dukakis, who had been a frequent guest on the morning show at BZ, had asked me to work on his campaign for Lieutenant-Governor in 1970. Fran Meaney, Michael's college roommate, was the campaign manager. I worked on all the radio and TV commercials for the campaign, helped recruit volunteers and wound up as a member of the candidate's "kitchen cabinet."

Michael got the Democratic nomination for Lieutenant-Governor that year, but as Kevin White's running mate, suffered the first major defeat of his political career. He was, as everyone knows by now, to suffer even bigger political set backs during the next twenty years. The biggest loss, of course, was the Presidential campaign of 1988.

In 1974, Michael ran successfully for Governor and, once again, I was proud to serve on his campaign team. We have remained close throughout the years.

The Meaneys and the Nolans grew to be good friends during the seventies. Our kids liked each other and we liked the Meaneys. Although we haven't seen Fran since the Meaneys divorced in the eighties, we still hold Pat's friendship as a special gift. She was there for us more than once during the management of Michele's illness.

In 1971, Michele and two year old Patrick and I spent the afternoon at the Jimmy Fund where Michele received her last treatment in this course of chemotherapy. Patrick, who was by now being called Packet, had been fussy all day. Normally a happy, jolly little fellow, I was a little concerned about his bad mood.

When we got back home I changed his diaper and noticed that he had

184

rash. A closer look and I discovered that what he had was a case of the Chicken Pox. I called Dr. Traggis.

"I'd like you to go straight over to Framingham General and have them give Michele a shot of gamma globulin, I'll call them and tell them you're coming. Then I want you to find a place where she can stay while the Chicken Pox runs its course through the family. It should be a place that's already had the disease," he told me.

Now, normally, Chicken Pox is not a concern for a healthy child, Michael, Traci and Teresa — along with little Patrick — would all become infected in the weeks ahead — and survive. Michele, however, was at great risk.

The Actinomycin-D had not only destroyed the cancer cells, but it had seriously depleted her immune system. A bout with Chicken Pox could make her very ill. In fact, Chicken Pox could even kill her. After all the odds we had seemingly overcome up to now, we sure as hell didn't want to lose her to a case of Chicken Pox.

There was only one possible solution. Michele would have to leave home until the disease had run its course through the family. That meant she would be gone for six weeks — at least. Teresa and the other kids had not, as yet, displayed any symptoms. They eventually would contract the disease, but right now our deep concern was in getting Michele away from the Pox.

That first night she was invited to stay with the the Cronin family, who lived one street away, but with Chicken Pox in the neighborhood, that was just too close to stay. We had to call on our new friends, again. And, of course, they all came through for us.

After that first night with my friend Linda Cronin, I packed my bags and hit the road. First, I was off to stay with our oldest New England friends, Charlie and Linda Austin. I probably would have spent the whole quarantine period with the Austins, but their oldest daughter, Lisa, came home from school with a fresh case of, you guessed it, Chicken Pox, at the end of two weeks. I was packed up and out of there in an hour.

My next stop was with the Jones of Carlisle. Judy Jones and Mom had worked together in Hawaii, before I was born. When Mom and Dad moved to New England they renewed their friendship.

Everyone likes Judy Jones. There were three Jones girls, one Teresa's age, one Patrick's age, and the middle one, Courtney, is my age. They had a lovely, contemporary home — a deck house — in the woods about ten miles from our house. I stayed there until the news came home on the bus that Chicken Pox had been discovered at school. That same afternoon, I was on the road, again. This time I headed to Pat and Fran Meaney's house in Brookline.

When I had spent six weeks away from home, the disease had run its course at our house, so I was allowed to come back. I sure did miss my family during the time I was away. Mom and Dad had been able to visit me, because they had both had Chicken Pox as children and weren't at risk of getting it again, or communicating it to me. But, after six weeks, I was sure anxious to get back to my room and my sisters and brothers who were now free of the normally harmless childhood disease of Chicken Pox.

Chicken Pox is a relatively unthreatening illness for most kids, but it's a disease that could have killed me.

As with the operations, the extended stay in the hospital after the brain surgery and all the trips to the clinic, Michele took the forced vacation from the family in stride. It wasn't really a big deal, so why make it a big deal? Her wonderful pragmatism has, I'm sure, made her life a lot easier than the lives many of us suffer through, worried about the things we can't change. If it can't be changed, Michele doesn't give it another thought. If, on the other hand, making a fuss can influence the outcome — stand back. I used to call her, "The Mobile Chain Saw." She could take you off at the knees if she caught you doing the wrong thing. No one, and I mean no one, wanted to suffer the wrath of Michele. It's the same way to this day in our family, Michele can be relentless.

It was about six months later, when the chemotherapy had been going for about two years that we were faced with a big decision. To continue the therapy or to discontinue it. Had we completely freed Michele of the very last bad cell in her body? If we stopped, would the cancer return? It was a difficult and important time in the management of Michele's disease.

One of our favorite doctors, the wonderful Dr. Demetrius Traggis, M.D., had been with Michele throughout the entire two years of treatment after the brain surgery. As we stood there, in the clinic, talking about what course we should take with the treatment he reminded me that Michele was the only child they could locate who had survived a Wilm's tumor of the brain. In fact, Dr. Traggis and three other members of the clinic team had written an article in the magazine, Pediatric Medicine, about Michele N., the only known survivor of a Wilm's cranial metastasis. He had given us a copy of the article.

"It's been two years. Is two years enough? Do we keep going? I just don't know what to recommend," he said.

"Maybe we should ask Michele what she thinks," I ventured.

Dr. Traggis looked a little stunned at my suggestion, but then said, "She's probably as good a judge of what we should do as anyone. Michele, what do you think we should do?"

I looked up at Mom and at this kind, wonderfully gentle man who had given so much to me and who had always held out the hope that one day we would get to this point. I know that my recovery had been a personal triumph for Dr. Traggis.

"Why don't we just stop everything?," I said.

"Well, it will probably be okay to stop, but there's always a chance that the cancer might not all be gone," Dr. Traggis told me.

"Don't worry. It's gone," I told him with complete confidence.

"I'd like to do a blood series on her every month for the next year and then regular exams every six month, if you don't mind," he said, knowing that his job was done — unless it turned out that I was wrong.

I know he was happy that I was doing so well, but I think Dr. Traggis also was a little sad that we would not be returning to The Jimmy Fund as regularly as we had been visiting for the past two years.

Dr. Traggis may have been a little sad that day, but my Mom had a big smile on her face when we left the Jimmy Fund. We went straight to the zoo to tell Dad that it was over.

Mom and Dad sat in the sun and cried a little, as they had lunch, while a skinny little kid with very, very short hair fed carrots to the Llamas.

He was always in too much
of a hurry to say, hello or how are you.
He just stormed in, did his thing — roughly — and stormed out.
He had hands like a teamster.
I hated seeing that guy come into the examining room.

Chapter Twelve

A Strange Twist!

In the fifth grade I failed an exam — an x-ray exam. The cancer had not returned, but the x-rays showed that I had developed a condition called scoliosis — curvature of the spine.

More new doctors, more new technicians and worst of all, more hassles were now in my future.

The orthopedic surgeon said that we had three choices: one, I could wear a back brace for about five years — or until my back stopped growing; two, I could have a couple of steel rods surgically implanted alongside my spine. After the operation I would be in a full body cast for six months; or three, I could do nothing and let my spine curve off toward New Hampshire.

Of course, I had to hear all this from my parents, not the doctor. Doctors never seem to clearly understand that the patient is also one of the people who need to be given the details of the situation — not just the parents. Even at eleven, I would have liked to have participated in the discussion. After all, the last time I checked, it was still my back.

After making my frustrations about being excluded from these doctor discussions known, things changed somewhat.

Mom and Dad would just tell whoever it was that wanted a private discussion that I was part of the team.

"Tell us all. We're all grownups here," Mom would say.

After that, I wasn't left out in the hall anymore.

Once, my Dad had an eminent radiologist on one of his magazine shows who talked, at length, about how the skeleton of a growing child is not just a small adult bone structure. Did you know that bones only grow from the ends, like flowers and trees?

After the show, Dad was able to spend some time with the doctor talking about the various effects of radiation on growth, digestion, soft tissue and the other delicate areas of a child's body.

We already knew that the therapeutic radiation I had been given after the brain surgery had damaged a lot of my otherwise normal brain cells. Even though they had taken great pains to direct the beams of radiation toward only the sight of the tumor, a lot of those rays penetrated healthy cells on the other side and in the surrounding brain tissue.

The damage those Roentgen of radiation did to the good brain cells would effect some, if not most, of my motor skills. For me, riding a bike came much later than for most kids. I am unable to coordinate the throwing of a ball with my right hand with the stride of my left foot. Sometimes I even throw left handed, because it doesn't really matter which hand I use, I throw so badly. The kind of coordination needed to throw out a runner in softball is not my long suit.

However, my normal, daily coordination is pretty good. I'm not awkward or clumsy. I walk just fine and I have fairly good balance, but when I run they can time me with a calendar. All of Jesse Owens' records are safe from Michele Nolan (and a lot of tortoise records, too).

As it turned out, the radiation had not only caused the scoliosis, but it had made my bones more brittle and less pliable. It was going to take a while to bring that curved spine back toward a straight position.

After some lengthy conversations about the pros and cons of each of the three courses of action, we all agreed — mostly Mom and Dad agreed, but at least I got to voice my fears and some of my concerns about those steel rods and the six years I would be strapped into a plastic body suit — that we'd take a few years in The Brace.

The Brace was developed at the medical centers in Boston. Childrens Hospital had — and still does have — one of the world's leading orthopedic units for growing bodies.

The head technician in the clinic, a guy named Mr. Miller, isn't one of the world's leading providers of TLC. I hated the way Mr. Miller behaved the first day I laid eyes on him.

He was, and still is, one of the country's foremost experts on correcting the long term effects of scoliosis. He also was, and I'm sure still is, one of the roughest people who ever put their hands on any part of my body. It was like having a gorilla push and twist and bend you.

He was also always in too much of a hurry to say Hello or How are you? He just stormed in, did his thing — roughly — and stormed out. He had hands like a teamster. I hated seeing that guy come into the examining room.

One of the other technicians, Bill Penny, was just the opposite. He was gentle and tender, with great hands. He always had time for a brief Hi, how are you today? Unfortunately, mine was such an exciting case that I almost always had to see the head guy, Mr. Miller.

They started the whole process of building a brace for me by wrapping me from my armpits to my thighs in plaster. Hot at first, then cold, clammy, wet plaster. I had to stand perfectly still for about thirty minutes while the plaster cast for the brace dried on my body.

Finally, old "rough hands" came in with a cutting tool and cut down both sides of the cast. They had their mold and I had a chapped, shriveled up, plaster splattered curved little body.

It took a few weeks to construct my brace. Mom took me in to have it fitted. Of course, old "rough hands" was waiting for me.

Actually, Mom and I were the ones who waited. We always waited for them in that unit. It didn't matter what time our appointment was, we always wound up cooling our heals in one of the semi-private little examining rooms, with me stripped to my underwear, for a half hour or more. The brace place was not my most favorite place to visit.

When they, at last, got the brace properly adjusted to Michele's body, they instructed me how to correctly put her into it. That's right, I didn't put it on Michele, I had to open the brace and insert the child.

It sounded cruel, at first, but after Michele was placed into the brace in the correct position, I had to pull the straps that held it together as tight as I could possible pull them. Michele usually had to hold onto a chair or another piece of furniture — or her sister — so that I didn't pull her across the room. The brace was one piece of special plastic — like the stuff hockey goalie masks are built from. The straps closed the braces' opening in the back and fastened with Velcro. The brace went from just under Michele's arms down to just where her hips bent. She could just sit while wearing the brace, which was good because she wore it for twenty-three hours every day, taking it off only for an hour each day to bath and apply lotion to her body.

As she did with everything else related to her "troubles," Michele soon adapted to wearing the brace, even at night. The major problem we had throughout the "battle of the brace" was finding things to wear under the brace which were light enough to allow the brace to do its work, yet thick enough to provide a cushion between her skin and the brace. The long series of tee shirts, cotton underwear and other things also had to fit fairly snugly around her tiny, misshaped body. Wrinkles were death. A wrinkle, pressed into her delicate flesh for twenty-three hours, always produced a painful, bright red welt. I had to be very careful and very patient whenever I put her into that brace.

Michele never complained about how tight we had to lace her into that thing. If I did leave it a little loose she would always say, "Tighter. If it's loose it rubs and pinches and hurts. Pull it real tight, Mom."

As Michele grew and as the brace began to correct the curve there had to be modifications made to the brace. When she outgrew one, we had to have another — bigger — one constructed.

Patsy normally took Michele into Boston to have her brace adjusted, but one time, when we were supposed to have a new brace, I offered to make the trip. I had heard the complaints about the long waits and the rough hands. I thought it might be of some help if I saw the situation for myself. Maybe I could help with an adjustment of my own. It turned out to be another of my adventures that might be called "Swimming up stream with Patrick in medicine land."

Dad made sure that we arrived at the clinic before it was time for our appointment. It wouldn't do to say something about the clinic keeping us waiting if we walked in late. As we parked the car, Dad made a special note of the time. We were ten minutes early.

We walked into the clinic about five minutes before our appointment. As I had been there on many previous occasions, the lady behind the desk greeted me by name.

"Hi, Michele. It will only be a few minutes." She always said exactly the same thing, "Hi Michele, it will only be a few minutes."

Dad and I sat down in the waiting room, but only for a few minutes. She always told the truth. We only waited there in the waiting room for a few minutes, but we waited in the examining area for hours.

Calling it a room is being extremely generous. It was just a draped off section of the big room. One of several little areas around the sides of the room which were each "kind of" draped off. Any pretense of privacy was ended whenever someone walked by or pulled open the drapes and just breezed in, so that anyone who wanted a look could see right into where one of us was sitting, usually half naked. I hated it.

Dad and I were alone in our little area for about fifteen minutes when Mr. Miller, breathless as usual, stuck his head through the curtain.

Now, understand, he and my Dad had never met.

Did he introduce himself? Did he say hello to Dad? No, to both questions. He just said to the room, "It's going to be a while longer," as his head disappeared.

Dad, still calm, pulled back the curtain. Mr. Miller was halfway across the big room by now.

"Excuse me, Miller, isn't it?"

"Yes, that's right."

"How much longer will it be then, Mr. Miller?," Dad asked, very politely.

"Why don't you go get a cup of coffee," Mr. Miller suggested.

"Mr. Miller, I didn't ask you what I should do with the time. I asked you how long it was going to be," Dad said, firmly.

"It's probably going to be a good half hour or so," Miller said, starting to walk away.

My Dad, still calm, but now moving into some of his favorite territory said, "Excuse me, Mr. Miller, but I don't have an extra half hour to wait while you do your job."

Mr. Miller turned back toward Dad as my Father now commanded the attention of everyone in the entire clinic.

"You made this appointment over two weeks ago, Mr. Miller," Dad reminded him. "We agreed, when this appointment was made, that I would have Michele here, on time, to be fitted with her new brace and you agreed, by making this appointment, that you would have your brace here. I'm here and obviously so is Michele. I've held up my part of the bargain. Where's your brace, Mr. Miller?"

"We need to make a few more adjustments."

"You've had two weeks to make those adjustments, Mr. Miller." Miller was trapped.

"Now you're asking us to sit here, cooling our heels or going for coffee while you do what you've had two weeks to do. I'm not prepared to give you thirty more minutes of our time while Michele and I sit here and wait for you to do what you should have done before we got here."

"Then I guess you'll have to come back. When would be a good time?," Mr. Miller asked, looking for a way to end this embarrassing encounter.

"You tell me when you'll have that brace ready for Michele to try on and I'll have her here at that time. It's completely up to you, Mr. Miller," Dad told him.

"Then come back one week from today. Same time."

"That will be fine, but, Mr. Miller, I want to be sure we understand each other. I'll have Michele here a week from today. You have your brace here, ready to be fitted."

"We'll be ready," Miller said as he walked from the room.

I got dressed and we left the clinic, but our exciting day wasn't quite over yet.

When we got to the parking garage we found the car and drove to the cashier's booth.

"That'll be $6 bucks," said the attendant, as he time stamped the ticket.

"It's only $3.00. We've been here exactly one hour," said Dad.

"An hour and ten minutes."

"Not true."

Dad's blood was still hot from the episode with Mr. Miller.

"I know the exact time we drove in and I know the exact time now," Dad said as he pulled the car over to the side so that if someone else wanted to pay and leave the garage, they could. Dad asked me to stay put, in the car. But we had a Mustang convertible, with the top down, so I could hear the whole thing.

Walking back to the little booth, Dad told the attendant that he knew the exact time we had entered the parking garage because being on time for the appointment had been a very important item.

"It was nine fifty when I drove in and got my ticket. When you stamped that ticket, just now, it was ten forty seven, that's less than an hour and I'm only paying for parking for an hour in your garage, Pal."

"It was nine forty when you pulled in, it's right here on the back of your ticket. See?," returned the attendant.

"No way," said Dad reaching into his pocket and pulling out a slip of paper. "Time stamp this piece of paper with your little exit machine there."

"Why?," asked the attendant.

"Because we're going to compare clocks, Pal. Now stamp the time on this piece of paper."

The guy didn't want to do it, but he couldn't come up with a quick reason why he shouldn't, so he put the piece of paper into the time clock and the clock stamped it, clunk. Dad took the paper out of his hand and walked over to the entrance, which was only a few feet from the booth. In a few seconds the next car drove into the garage and the automatic machine punched out a parking ticket for the driver.

Dad said the the driver, "Excuse me, we're checking the clocks. May I see that for just one second, please?"

"Sure," the lady said, looking only a little puzzled.

"Very interesting, my friend. Who sets these clocks?," Dad asked.

"I do," said the attendant.

"Well, the piece of paper you punched less than a minute ago in your exit booth says ten forty nine. This ticket says the time is, ten thirty five. You've got these clocks set fourteen minutes apart. I'll bet you pick up more than a few extra dollars that way.

"Nice try, but you lose, Pal," Dad said, handing the guy the three dollars we owed for parking.

193

"But I've already rung up six dollars," the guy protested.

"Then I suggest you pony up the other three dollars unless you want to be short. You just told me that you're the guy who sets these clocks."

Dad winked at me as we drove out of the parking garage. He was two for two that day and it had been a very interesting morning for a fifth grader.

The next week when we returned to the clinic — once again, on time — the brace and Mr. Miller were both waiting for us. The guy in the parking garage was new and the clocks were correctly set.

Oh, yeah, Dad checked them.

During the next few months, Michele wore her brace throughout the day and night, each morning, taking it off to bathe and get ready for school. It became a very routine matter for both her and the rest of the family.

Each morning I would leave for work with the three middle school kids, Michele, Traci and Michael. Usually, Jennifer Schultz, another eleven year old who was best friends with both Michele and Traci, would join us. Jennifer lived just two doors away. I dropped them all off at school as I went through the town center.

Taking them to school meant that they didn't have to wait in the cold by the side of the road for the school bus. I was always worried that some driver might slip on the icy road and hit one of them as they waited at the bus stop. The Town of Sudbury didn't plow the sides of the narrow town roads very well when it snowed.

On the eleventh of January, a huge storm dumped over three feet of snow on Middlesex County that year. The road crews had been out all night plowing and sanding the streets and roads.

When the morning dawned, bright and clear but with snow piled high along all the roads in town, I knew I didn't want the kids standing at the edge of the road waiting for a bus.

Normally, Michele was always given the passenger seat because the brace made it uncomfortable for her to climb into the back seat of the Mustang. However, on this particular morning, Jennifer was late so Michele just eased into the back seat with Traci. It meant that when Jennifer got there she could just slip in and we could go. Which she did, a few minutes later.

We turned onto Horse Pond Road, stopping a few houses down to pick up another of the kids' classmates, a little girl named Chris Brown.

Since the front seat was full, Michael was sitting next to me and Jennifer was in the passenger seat, Chris slipped into the back seat with Traci and Michele. Michele was sitting in the middle. Traci was behind me.

There is, in the Town of Sudbury, a very dangerous intersection where Peakham Road and Union Avenue come together. It had been the scene of several crashes and near crashes over the years. Both are country roads, without center lines or much of a shoulder. Peakham Road, the one we were driving on, did not have a stop sign at that intersection, but Union Avenue did. However, the trees and shrubs and the way the road rose as Peakham Road came to the intersection, made it extremely difficult to see traffic approaching from the left. A driver coming up Union, who had stopped, had to ease out almost into Peakham Road before he could see if it was safe to proceed. Extreme caution needed to be taken with this corner by all drivers.

As both roads were heavily traveled at this time of the day, I was always very careful at this junction. I approached at a safe speed and then would ease off the accelerator and just coast through, watching for any cars that might be edging out, particularly from the right.

On this particular morning I was even more cautious than usual because the snow banks were so high along all sides of all the roads. Seeing down the road to the right, before you were actually in the intersection, was impossible since the snow bank at the corner was over ten feet high.

I eased up to the corner, I glanced to the left and then looked to the right. Seeing no cars, I let the Mustang continue through the intersection, coasting at about fifteen miles an hour. Just at we were in the middle of the intersection I saw that a car was right on top of us, bearing down at an alarming speed. The driver hadn't stopped, easing out into the intersection to see if it was clear, he was speeding right through the intersection. He was running through the stop sign. He was going to hit us — hard.

I clearly remember that for just an instant I experienced a overpowering feeling of frustration. It was not fear I felt, but total frustration, knowing that we were going to be hit by this speeding car and knowing that there wasn't a single thing I could do about it. I didn't have time to warn the kids or to take any action — crash, in a millisecond the huge car crashed into the side of our Mustang, right at the passenger door.

The sounds of broken glass and metal scraping on metal seemed to last for an hour, as our car was slammed across the intersection and into the snow bank on the opposite side of the road. When we finally stopped, the car that hit us was still against the side of our car. I guess the guy had completely missed the fact that this was a cross street. He apparently didn't even see the snow covered stop sign. Being from another town, he was rushing to work on a strange road and suddenly, without warning, a little white Mustang filled with eleven year olds popped up right in front of him.

There were no skid marks, no signs of any braking action on his part. In the police report he stated that he stopped at the stop sign and then, as he attempted to start up, the wheels spun on the ice, suddenly catching and propelling his car into the intersection.

In truth, had he been stopped or even just moving, I would have seen him or he would surely have seen us before starting up. In truth, if he had stopped, spun his tires, had them suddenly grab and then hit us, I doubt his car would have had the power to slam us across the road, jam us into a snow bank, bounced off and come to rest only a foot or so from the demolished door of the Mustang.

I'll always believe that he just didn't know he was approaching an intersection. In his rush to get to work, he had not been paying as careful attention on a snow banked country road, as he should have been.

When the noise finally stopped Traci was the first one to speak. "Dad, what happened?"

"That guy hit us, Honey. Don't anyone move. Just sit still, you might be hurt and not realize it. Does anyone seem to be hurt back there?"

I turned to look in the back and I could see that they were all still conscious. Looking back at me from the darkness in the rear seat were six of the biggest eyes I have ever seen. Traci was bleeding from a cut on the side of her face.

"Honey, you're bleeding," I said to Traci. "But it doesn't look like any more than a scratch. Just sit tight. I've got to see about Jen."

Michael was laying against me, completely unconscious. He had no signs of injury, and he was breathing, so I didn't think he was in any immediate danger. Jennifer was also unconscious, but she was bleeding all over the front seat. I had to see to her right away.

A face suddenly appeared where the passenger window had been. It was the face of the driver of the car that hit us.

"Is everyone all right?," he asked.

"No!," I told him. "Everyone is not all right. Get over to that house and call the police. Tell them that we have five injured children here and we need medical attention immediately."

He turned and ran toward the house on the corner, leaving his car where it had come to rest only a foot from our car, blocking the intersection.

I couldn't see how badly Jennifer was hurt from where I was. There was an unconscious Michael and three sets of winter clothes between us. I'd have to get out of the car and go around to the other side before I could attend to Jennifer's injuries, but my door was jammed up against a huge snow bank. I couldn't crawl over the two unconscious kids. I was trapped, but I knew I had to reach Jennifer as quickly as possible. She might be bleeding to death.

Fortunately I was driving a convertible, so I simply released the latches which held the top to the windshield and pulled the knob that lowered the top. As soon as I had enough room to climb out over the windshield, I did so.

By now several other motorists had stopped to help. One of them was Traci's teacher.

"How can I help?," she asked.

"Help me see how badly Jennifer is hurt. But let's be very careful," I said, "She looks badly injured."

Jennifer had long blond hair. It was all over her face and head, stained red with her blood. I thought she might already be dead.

Gently, the teacher and I pulled back the hair from Jennifer's face and neck. I felt for a pulse in her neck. I was greatly relieved to find a strong pulse. Jennifer was still alive. The blood was all coming from a thousand tiny cuts on the back of her ear and side of her neck. There wasn't any big, deep wound, just a lot of little bleeding cuts from flying glass. I relaxed a little.

"She doesn't seem to be sitting just right," the teacher said.

"She may have injured her neck. We took quite a shot from the side," I said.

At that moment, the guy who hit us returned.

"There isn't anyone home at that house," he said.

I quickly realized that the man was suffering from shock and was not able to think or act clearly.

"Then go to another house," I told him.

"Can I help?," asked another man who appeared as if from nowhere.

"Yes. Drive down the the police station. It's just there at the bottom of the hill. Tell them we need an ambulance up here for injured children," I instructed him. He jumped into his car and sped away.

"What can I do?," asked another motorist.

"Go get my wife. We live just down the road. Twenty-one Stonebrook. Do you know where Stonebrook Road is?"

"Yes. I know Stonebrook," he said.

"We're the fourth house on the left. Just bring her here. Her name's Patsy."

I was just getting Patrick dressed when I heard a loud banging on the front door and a voice calling my name.

"Come around to the side door. The front door is frozen shut," I shouted.

I went out through the kitchen and family room to meet whoever had been pounding on the door at our side door, the one that opened.

"Can you come with me right away? Your husband has been in a traffic accident and he sent me to get you," the man said.

"Of course. Is he all right?"

"He's got a little cut on his face, but he seems to be okay."

"What about the kids?," I demanded.

"I don't know anything about the kids," he said.

Was he lying? Were the kids hurt or dead? Was he trying not to panic me? If he was, he wasn't don't a very good job.

"Packet," I instructed the seven-year-old. "You run over to Dickie's house. Tell him that I said you were to stay with him until I get back. It may be a while. I'll take you to school when I get home."

"Come on," I said to the stranger who had been sent to fetch me. "Let's go."

Grabbing my coat and gloves, we were out the door.

As we drove away from the house the man told me that the accident was at Peakham and Union and that the car was badly damaged, but that Patrick was out of the car and was giving instructions. He said Patrick just wanted me brought there as quickly as possible. I was sure that one or more of the kids was dead or at the very least, badly damaged. I hoped with all my heart that it wasn't Michele.

I leaned behind Jennifer and into the back seat to check more carefully on the three kids back there. They were being so very good. They were just sitting there, waiting for me to tell them what to do next. No crying, no fussing. Michele had given Traci a tissue to hold to her facial cut. All three seemed to be otherwise uninjured.

"Don't move, kids. Help will be here soon and we'll get you out, but the safest place for you is right where you are." They all just nodded..

In just a few minutes, police cars and fire engines arrived from all directions. I think they must have scrambled every unit in town. It's a quiet town, not much exciting ever happens there, so we got the full treatment.

"Please step back, sir," one of the firemen instructed me as he started

197

to push me aside.

"Hold it, pal. Let's not start ripping kids out of that car. Some of them are hurt," I said.

"Are you a doctor?," he demanded to know.

"No, but I'm a Father. Those are my kids and I want you to be very careful and not go all gung ho here."

"It's all right," said another, calmer, young fireman. "We're all EMTs. We know what we're doing."

"Okay. Just go easy. We're not on fire, everyone's breathing, so just take your time."

I stepped back a few feet to let the emergency workers have access to Jennifer.

As they placed a cervical collar around her neck and a hard board behind her back, one of the policemen walked over to me and handed me a bandage.

"Here," he said. "Better use this on your face."

"Why?," I asked.

"'cause you're bleeding."

I didn't even know I'd been cut. As it turned out, Michael had probably been knocked unconscious when his head banged against mine. He was out cold, I was cut and bleeding.

"Thanks," I said to the cop.

"Doesn't look too serious. Just a scratch. You doing all right, otherwise?," he asked.

"Yeah. I think so. I've had a couple of broken ribs which were just starting to heal. I think I may have reinjured them, that's all."

My back was starting to tighten up as I stood there in the cold. It was the first time since the crash that I had even stopped to take any kind of a personal inventory. My back and side were now beginning to ache.

"Better have the Doc check it out, after he fixes that cut," he told me.

"Thanks. I will. Thanks for coming so quickly."

"Just doing our job."

As we drove up to the scene of the accident, all I could see were fire trucks and cop cars. Red and blue lights were flashing everywhere. I could see Patrick standing in the middle of the road talking to one of the Sudbury policemen. I jumped out of the truck, thanked the guy who had come to get me, and ran over to Patrick.

"What happened, Honey? Are you alright?"

"A guy ran the stop sign and t-boned us. I only saw him a second before he hit us. There wasn't anything I could do."

"What about the kids?," I asked, wanting to know, afraid to hear.

"Michael's out cold, but I don't think he's hurt badly. Traci and Michele seem to be OK. Traci's got a cut on her face. Chris Brown is OK."

"You picked up Chris, too."

"Sure. It's cold out here. But it's Jennifer that I'm really worried about.. She's unconscious. The back of her neck and her right ear are cut in a million places. I think her neck might be hurt too. That damn car hit us right on Jen's door. And just look at what it did to the car, Babe" Patrick said.

"Poor Jen. I'm going to see if I can help."

By now Michael was partially awake. He was able to get out of the car under his own power, but he didn't know where he was or what day it was. I put him in the front seat of one of the police cars.

Jennifer had been carefully removed from the front seat of the car and was placed on a stretcher in the ambulance. The firemen put a tarp over the kids in the back seat and just pulled the soft top of the car back away from them. It made it easier to get them out. They were all able to walk to a waiting police car.

"Are we going to school, Dad?", Traci asked.

"No, honey. We're all going to the hospital. The doctors are going to check everyone over to make sure we're okay. You ride with Mom and Michele and me," I told her.

"Okay."

As Patsy and I got into the front seat, Michele, Chris and Traci got into the back seat of the police car.

Since Sudbury doesn't have a hospital, we were all taken to Framingham General, in the next town. On the way, one of our friends, a woman who had been a teacher, at one time or another, to all five of the kids in the accident, sat in traffic, waiting to turn. Missy Stuefloten was headed to school to teacher her class. She saw me in the front seat of the police car. Missy just switched her turn indicator to the other side and followed us to the hospital, instead of going to school.

When we got to the hospital Patsy turned her full attention to Jennifer. As they went to x-ray, one of the technicians told Patsy that she would have to wait outside.

"Sorry. I'm not going to have her wake up, not knowing where she is, surrounded by strangers. It's bad enough that she's been hurt. We don't have to scare her anymore than she's already going to be. You do your job, and I'll do mine," said Patsy in a way that left no room for debate. The discussion was over. Together they wheeled Jen into x-ray to see just how badly she was broken.

I went around to each of the kids to see how they were. I insisted that the doctor get every child undressed, even if they seemed to be fine.

"Mr. Nolan, we need to take care of your facial injury. The kids will be fine," said a nurse.

"I'll be right back, guys. Just take it easy and tell the doctor what he needs to know. If something hurts, tell him."

The nurse took me into a trauma room where a young doctor was preparing the things he needed to sew up my wounds. I must have looked like I'd lost a fight with Ali.

While I was getting stitched up, one of the nurses came in and said, "Doctor, can you let Mr. Nolan come with me for just a second. His son Michael is a little more awake now and he's worried about his dad. He thinks we're just telling him that Dad's okay. He's afraid his dad is really badly injured."

"I'll be right back," I told them, not waiting for the doctor to reply.

Michael was laying on a gurney in the hallway. He was very confused and still a little out of it. He was sure that I was either hurt badly or dead.

He was also a little scared. He didn't know where he was. I told him I was fine and that everything was going to be okay. Just relax and rest, I told him. He laid back, much more at ease, but still a little punch drunk.

It took eleven stitches to repair the cuts Michael's head had opened on my face.

The Doctor and I took a look at Jennifer's x-rays, together. It was clear that she had been the most seriously injured of the children. There on the x-ray plate you could clearly see that both of her collarbones were broken. She also had three broken ribs.

"I don't think she's sustained any trauma to her neck, but I'd like the radiologist to take a look at her cervical study," the doctor said.

"It does look like she's going to have a tough time raising either arm for a few days," I said. "Poor kid. What about her cuts?"

"I think we'll wait until she wakes up before we start to suture them. I don't think we should be working on her when she comes around," he said.

"She's been making some sounds and she seems to be coming out of it a little," I told him.

"She's going to have hell of a headache, too. Has anyone called her parents?"

"I don't think so. Why don't we ask Patrick."

We wheeled Jennifer out of x-ray and back into the emergency room. Patrick and our friend, Missy Stuefloten, the kid's teacher who had followed us to the hospital, were talking with a nurse about Jennifer.

"Jennifer has just recently lost her father to cancer. I didn't think it's a good idea to call Jean and tell her that Jennifer has been injured in a car wreck. One of us should go get Jean," I suggested.

"I'll go," said Missy. "I know her. She knows me and it's something that I can do to help. I'll bring her back as soon as I can."

Missy turned and ran to her car. It was a wonderful thing for her to do for us. At a time like this everyone always asks, what can I do to help? Here was something that could be done that was very helpful. Thanks, Missy.

I wanted to make sure that each of the kids had been carefully examined by the doctors and the nurses. Chris Brown, Traci and Michele were being held in an examining room in the rear of the emergency area. I walked in as the doctor was finishing his examination of Traci. They had already repaired the cuts she had sustained on the side of her face.

"How's the head, Traci?"

"It's okay, Dad. It didn't even hurt too much to get the stitches."

"Brave girl," I said, giving her a hug. "But, remember, Michele is still way ahead on stitches. Everything else OK?"

"She seems to be fine. A little tender on one side, but I think it's just a bump from an elbow. I think the fact that these three were packed in so tightly in the back seat helped keep them from being tossed around in the car and getting hurt. Chris here is fine, too," said the doctor.

"What about Michele?," I asked.

"I was just getting to her when you came in. Michele, let's slip off your dress and take a look."

Traci unbuttoned Michele's dress in the back and I pulled it off over

200

her head. When the dress came off, Michele's brace fell on the floor in two pieces. The force of the impact had broken the brace in half, right down the front.

"What's this?," asked the doctor.

"She has scoliosis. It's her back brace, but it's supposed to be in one piece," I said.

"Looks like she had a little extra protection back there. If the crash broke this stuff," he said examining the brace as he picked it up, "It's lucky for Michele that she was wearing it."

"Most days she would disagree with you about being lucky to have to wear it, but today, I think she might not."

I was certainly happy she was wearing it. I was also happy that Jennifer had been late, even though it meant that she had not been in the back seat where she normally rode, but instead, had been in the front seat where she suffered the most damage. You see, if Michele and her brace had been in that front seat, the crash might very well have killed her. While the brace helped Michele survive the impact of the crash while wedged between the other two girls in the back seat, in the front seat, against the door that the car hit, that same brace might have prevented her from bending and she might have broken. While it was a tragic day for us all, it could have been a lot worse, especially for Michele.

It was just another time when Michele was in the path of near death, but was able to dodge the bullet.

For three years, Michele had been "zapped"
with hundreds of Roentgen of radiation,
all during her primary growing period,
causing damage to her spine, her intestines,
her lungs and to her general growth plates.

Chapter Thirteen

Survival Can Be Tough On A Girl!

When those to whom you trust your health — even your survival — tell you that without a series of painful and damaging radiation treatments you will probably not survive the attack of the cancer cells which have invaded your body, you don't even think about side effects.

As Patrick says, "You just march off to the x-ray department and climb up on the table."

When your hair falls out, you get a wig. When your appetite disappears and your body is just skin and bones, you make black jokes about Weight Watchers, starving children, World War II prison camps and falling through a hole in the seat of your own pants. At the time you're battling the disease, your only concern is the process of survival — period.

For three years, Michele had been "zapped" with hundreds of Roentgen of radiation, all during her primary growing period, causing damage to her spine, her intestines, her lungs and to her general growth plates.

As a three-year-old, they had blasted the site of the original tumor in her abdomen. Her lungs had been irradiated. That one spot in her left lung had been heavily zapped. Her brain had received more of the deadly rays than probably were needed; we'll never know. What we do know is, after twenty plus years, it's beginning to look like she didn't received too few Roentgen. She's still with us.

The radiation to her stomach and chest went right through to her back and severely reduced the proper growth in portions of her spine, developing in it a severe case of scoliosis.

The radiation also slowed the overall growth of her spine and she was only able to grow to a final height of four feet nine and one half inches.

The same damaging doses of radiation cooked the left lob of Michele's liver, severely reducing its productivity. The rays caused a constriction in her small intestine which required another major surgery to correct when she was twenty-four years old.

One of the most emotionally damaging side effects didn't appear until Michele was around sixteen. The radiation to her chest had done terminal damage to the immature mammary gland in her left breast. That spot in her lung required a major, finely tuned series of high dose radiation treatments before it was eradicated. The general radiation to her chest caused the mammary glands to develop less than they might have without the radiation, but that triple dose to that recalcitrant spot slammed the brakes on any growth at all for the left side.

As the rest of Michele's body grew into a young woman, that left mammary gland remained dormant. Even though the right side only developed minimally, the left side didn't even bud. We had her fitted for a prosthetic device that slid comfortably into a pocket in her bra. I sewed a pouch into her swimming suits so that she was always balanced, even while swimming.

Even though I'm sure that no one ever bothered to notice that she was lopsided, in her mind, Michele believed that everyone knew that she was "different," abnormal, a freak.

She would wear long sleeved shirts and blouses, even on hot days. She would only wear high collared shirts and never, ever, a tee shirt, except when she went swimming and then she wore a tee short over her swim suit. In her mind, she knew that everyone was staring at a poor, deformed girl, who had only one breast.

She started to wear her bras to bed at night. She cut back on bathing because it meant getting completely undressed, even though she bathed in private.

Finally, she became reluctant to even leave the house. She didn't want us to entertain. Here was a young teenager quickly withdrawing into a safe, protected world where she could be seen only by her family. Even that world was retreating to the point where she wouldn't disrobe in front of her mother or her sisters anymore.

The problem was growing further and further out of proportion each day, in Michele's mind. It didn't help to say that it was just in Michele's mind. We were facing yet another problem that had to be dealt with as straightforwardly as possible, just as we had dealt with all the other problems.

Patrick and I sent all of the other kids to the park one day so we could sit down with Michele to talk about some solutions to the problem, without any unnecessary interruptions.

Michele was reluctant to even discuss this serious and growing problem with her parents. She wanted to just block it out, push it to the back of her mind and stay in the house. She did not want to address the issue in any way, all the while seeming to dwell more and more heavily on it in her own mind. We were nearing the threshold of a serious psychological problem here and we both knew it. Something had to be done.

"Michele," I said, "Dad and I want to talk about your undeveloped breast. We know it's going to be difficult to talk about because you're so private about how you feel, but, honey, we have to talk about it."

"This is a discussion just between the three of us, no one else will know anything about what we talk about here, unless you want them to know," Patrick assured her.

"I don't want to talk about it, dad," she said in an annoyed tone, starting, even with just the mention of the discussion, to get upset.

Tears came to her eyes as she spoke. She began to choke up. Here was a kid who had been able to meet the devil head on, look him in the eye and stare him down, but who was ashamed and scared to talk to her mother and father about an undeveloped breast and what might be done to correct it. It was time to push a little.

"We really don't have any choice, baby. We have to talk about it. You don't want to go anywhere, you don't want anyone to come over to the house. You want to stay in your room all day. We've got to deal with it," Patrick said quietly, but firmly.

"We know that the little false breast we got for you isn't doing what it should be doing for you, but we have a suggestion about what can," I said.

"What?," she demanded impatiently, through the tears, still rejecting the discussion, but now accepting, as she always has at such times, that she really had no choice.

"There's a simple surgical procedure that they can do where they just take a little bag of silicone and slip it inside, under the skin," Patrick told her.

"Well, it's actually not the very one you've been wearing, but it's just like it. In fact it can be one that's even more like your right breast than this one is."

"Really? They can really do that, mom?" She started to brighten a bit.

"Really. All they do is make a very small incision under here." I indicated on my own breast, "Then they insert a small package of silicone gel. No more pockets in your bras, no more pouches in the swim suits and no more embarrassment about being different than the other girls."

"But who does this? You know I don't want just anyone doing something like this to me, mom."

Two years previously, during Michele's freshman year in high school, we had moved from Sudbury to Reno, Nevada, leaving all of her trusted doctors behind, three thousand miles away on the East Coast. I had accepted a position as the Charge Nurse in the Telemetry Department at Washoe Medical Center, the area's regional hospital. I knew most of the doctors in town.

Patrick said, "I'll tell you what we do. You get mom to give you a list of the best plastic surgeons in town. Then you call them up and make an appointment to talk to them. Tell their appointment secretary, on the phone, that you don't want to be examined, you just want ten minutes of the doctor's time to talk to him, to interview him for a job. Time for which you're willing to pay. Then, go interview them, pick out the guy you like. If there isn't one you like here in Reno, we'll go to San Francisco and do the same thing until we find a doctor you're comfortable with."

Working at Washoe Medical Center, I knew — or knew of — every one of the city's plastic surgeons. I called the OR nurse to ask her advice on whom she thought was the best we could get for Michele. She gave me three names. I passed those names on to Michele. The first one she called was the guy who had been given the highest recommendation by all those I talked to at the hospital when I asked around about plastic surgeons.

Michele wanted to go to the appointment alone. I was proud of her, because I knew it was taking a lot of courage for her to do this, but I also knew how badly she wanted to be as physically normal as she possible could be.

After the appointment with the first guy, Patrick and I talked with her about the visit. This time she was completely relaxed and ready to have a talk about her breast implant.

"He's a real nice man, dad. I'll let him do it, if we don't find someone I like better. But, dad, the guy's so fat that he has to kind of lean on a stool. He can't even sit on it. If a guy doesn't care any more about himself then that, how can I be sure he'll care about me and my body?"

"You can't. Who's next on the list?," Patrick said.

"A guy who's name I can't even pronounce," she laughed. It had been a while since she had laughed about this particular subject. At that moment it was evident to both Patrick and I that the healing had already begun.

"John Iliescu," I said. "They tell me he's really good and really good with his patients."

"Well, I'm calling him tomorrow," she said flatly, heading off to bed.

"I think we're doing a very smart thing here," I said to Patrick.

"I think you're brilliant, that's what I think," he said, kissing me.

A few days later Michele gave us the report on John Iliescu.

"Dad, this guy's a real person. He sat on the table beside me, instead of standing or sitting across the room on a stool. He treats you like you're a person, not a patient." She was filled with enthusiasm.

"Sounds like you've got your man, honey," I said.

"He's great," she said, more like a young lady talking about a new boyfriend than a patient talking about her plastic surgeon.

Appointments were made, blood tests were drawn, schedules were completed and before long the day was finally at hand.

This type of breast augmentation is a very simple procedure, with the patient barely unconscious. It is done as an out-patient or, same day, surgical procedure.

The morning of the surgery, we all assembled in the out-patient lounge, waiting for the orderly who would come to take Michele to surgery. Traci was there and, with a screaming migraine headache, so was Teresa. Our son Patrick had chosen to go to school. He knew he was hopelessly outnumbered in that group.

As it turned out, Patsy and I were unneeded window dressing, too. This was Michele's day. She was queen of all she surveyed. She had her caring doctor waiting to make her normal. She had her two sisters with her as a loving court of attendants. Mom and I were just there to drive her home when it was all over.

She was only in the OR for about forty minutes before they brought Michele back to the out-patient surgery area to recover from the anesthesia. By the time she got back to us she was already awake. Groggy, but awake and aware.

"It's all over, sweetie," Patsy told her.

"Really? It's done?"

"As soon as you're completely awake we can go home. How do you feel?"

"I feel great. That stuff they give you is really terrific," she smiled. It was a wicked smile …wickedly.

"It's not something you want to get used to," Patrick said.

Later, Michele told us that in the operating room, before they put her to sleep, Dr. Iliescu had come in to tell her that he knew how privately she felt about her body. He said he wanted her to know that he was there to protect and preserve her dignity. No one, he said, no one, would make fun of her, laugh at her or in anyway be unkind, even after she was asleep.

This guy Iliescu should have been in public relations or politics. That day, he made a friend and a follower, for life. For Michele, he could walk on water.

In the next few weeks an amazing transformation took place within our young lady. Michele stopped hiding in her room. She started sleeping in a tee shirt, without a bra. She started to return to the old, outgoing, friendly Michele that we had all known and loved.

Within a few weeks, you couldn't believe it was the same young lady. Michele was no longer "different" or malformed.

I'll always be completely amazed at the difference between the teenage Michele with just one breast and the Michele who appeared when she finally had two.

During our three year stay in Reno Michele gained a new breast, graduated from Reno High School — amid tears of joy from her whole family — and we lost Michael.

During his freshman year in high school, Michael developed some radical, and frightening, changes in his personality. It was due, we now believe, to a condition known as Fetal Alcohol Syndrome. That's when the unborn child, in this case Michael, is severely affected by the drinking of the birth mother. They say that all the clues were there for us to see; the poor vision, the dyslexia, the desire to please as a youngster followed by the near sociopathic behavior that develops as a teenager. All the symptoms of FAS were there in Michael. Tragically, his brain was terribly damaged even before he was born.

In 1984, Michael was arrested on two counts of felony arson. He had, on two consecutive nights, attempted to burn down our home. After months of court appearances, lawyers, in-patient psychiatric care and tens of thousands of dollars, Michael, with our permission, was emancipated by the State of Nevada. Seven months short of his eighteenth birthday, Michael was legally allowed to accept full responsibility for himself, as an adult.

He broke off all contact and communication with the family. He was only seen twice briefly by any of us after that; first by Traci, who had a very brief chance encounter with him at a local convenience store in 1988 and by Teresa who in 1993 saw his picture in the paper and sought him out for a visit. They enjoyed a long and very fruitful chat.

On March 21, 1994, six months after that "good" visit with Teresa and one month after his twenty-eighth birthday, Michael was discovered shot to death in Phoenix, Arizona. The police believe he had been the victim of a bad drug deal. In his early twenties, Michael had been incarcerated for three years on drug dealing charges and was known to the Phoenix police as a member of the local drug scene.

Michael's death brought to a close a sad chapter in our lives. A chapter that started out hopefully, followed by fourteen wonderful years.

That wonderful, bright beginning was followed by fourteen years of sadness, pain and a terrible void.

It can be said that all during the early years of Michele's treatment, Michael was a loyal and trusted brother who stood by her and worried about her, continually.

There rests within each of us in our family a private emptiness that, in my case, will haunt me for the rest of my days, because we recognize that while we were able to save Michele from her cancer, we were unable to rescue Michael from his private demons.

Another side effect of her treatment developed a couple of years later when she was in college. Something in the back of her head had started to cause a tenderness in her scalp. It wasn't a pain, but it was something sharp under the skin that made her head sore whenever the pillow or a chair cushion touched that part of her scalp.

An x-ray was taken which showed a tiny wire, probably one of the wires used to hold in place the piece of skull they had removed for the brain surgery years before, just under the skin. It had worked its way up through the softened bone to the surface and was "sticking" her from the inside. The radiation, of course, had caused that part of her skull to be softer and more porous than normal skull bone.

In another out-patient procedure, this time in Los Angeles under a local anesthesia, a neurosurgeon removed the wire. After the surgery we learned that this particular surgeon had been one of the young medical school students who, eighteen years before in Boston, had been a member of the surgical team the day Larry Page locked the operating room and removed that brain tumor from Michele's head.

Now, three thousand miles away from that operating room, a doctor in Los Angeles had written the final chapter to that medical report. Small world.

When I was a teenager, starting to have menstrual periods, I realized that my monthly cycles would actually only appear once every other month. It seems, the doctors told us, that the radiation to the left side of my abdomen had, unfortunately, hit my tiny left ovary with full force. The rays of the radiation treatments had apparently completely destroyed that ovary. I am only running on one reproductive cylinder. It was, however, kind of a treat to only have six periods a year, instead of the twelve that my sisters had to deal with.

It does scare me a little bit that the one ovary which does function might also have been damaged by the radiation. If it has been affected, I may not be able to get pregnant, but we won't know about that until the day comes when I'm ready to have a child.

However, my sister, Teresa and I have had a discussion about the possibility that I might not be fertile. Teresa says that if I can't conceive a child on my own, she will give me one of her eggs which can be fertilized, in vitro, and then implanted in my womb. It's nice to have a thoughtful big sister to look out for you.

My two sisters, Teresa and Traci — like my Mom and Dad — have always been there for me. My sisters and my brother Patrick are my three very best and closest friends.

The radiation treatments also fried a large portion of my liver and did some serious damage to the top portion of my small intestine. We knew, through liver function tests, that for a while I was running at maximum capacity on my liver, but we didn't find out about how serious the damage had been to the small intestine until I was twenty-four.

I was never a very big eater, although I do love food. It was just that I would feel full long before my plate was empty.

Some time after my twenty- fourth birthday, in June of 1989, I started to notice that I continued to experience the feeling of having just eaten a large meal hours after I had actually finished eating. I was always a little bloated and uncomfortable.

Earlier that same spring, our family had moved to Whidbey Island, in Puget Sound, near Seattle where Mom went to work for Nordstrom as the company's Certified Occupational Health Nurse.

From a studio he and Patrick built in the new house, dad continued to work as a creative person and copywriter for several advertising agencies. A fax machine, his Macintosh computer and a daily visit from Federal Express allows Dad to work at home, most of the time. He does have to go into Seattle, or fly to Reno or LA from time to time to record commercials, but he's home almost all the time. It was during this time that he started work on this book.

Mom and Dad opened a golf driving range and I spent most of the summer handing out golf balls and driving the little tractor that picks up the balls. I had been looking for a job in a day care center, but I hadn't been able to find a position, as yet, during that summer. I knew that when school started in the fall, I would be able to find a good job with one of the child care centers, either on the island or just across Puget Sound on the mainland. There are dozens of centers within a fairly short commute of our house.

As summer drew to a close, fall turned the leaves gold and red. It's a lovely time of year on Puget Sound.

My plumbing, however, was not lovely. It had started to work less and less properly. Looking back, I don't think it ever really worked as it was supposed to work, but when I was twenty-four, it started to get really cranky.

I'd have days and days without experiencing a bowel movement, then I'd have near diarrhea for two days. I had a constant battle with gas and painful gas pains. The feeling of fullness, even when I hadn't eaten a thing for hours, reduced my intake. I was losing weight, losing strength and losing patience with this growing discomfort.

Michele has always been slow to complain. She just sticks out her chin and heads down the road when a pain or an ailment shows up. But, this time, we could tell that she was feeling poorly. She wasn't eating and her normal, rather outrageous, sense of humor was sagging. A very bad sign.

Within a few days, the intake was not only reduced to almost nothing, but the output was down to zero. A mild laxative reduced the gas in her stomach — somewhat — but had no real effect on the cranky intestinal tract.

A day later, when she woke up in the middle of the night sick to her stomach, it was time to seek medical attention. She could keep nothing in her stomach, not even a sip of water.

In a few hours she would begin to dehydrate, so off we went to the local island hospital.

Later that morning, mom checked me into Whidbey General, the island's only hospital, located about thirty miles north of our house in the small town of Coupeville. I was feeling very sick. My stomach was full of gas and I was getting weak from lack of nutrition. I knew I was in some serious distress, but I wasn't too scared. I didn't really think the cancer was back, but I did know that cancer was one of the possibilities — even after twenty years of being free of it. I also knew that mom and dad were on the case. They hadn't failed me before, so I had complete confidence in them and in their decisions about my health care.

It seems to me that someone in power always seems to give the delicate hospital jobs to those people with the heaviest hands. For all the IVs that I've had, only a few of them have been started by people who had any touch or feel for the job at all. Most of them are just jabbing in the needle, hoping to hit a vein. It takes a certain touch to do it right, even on normal veins. My veins are another story all together.

The chemotherapy and the radiation seriously damaged my veins. They're smaller, softer and they are not easy to find. It takes a skilled person to slip a needle into one of them. I always seem to get a beginner who is in need of a lot more practice.

At Whidbey General they wanted to get some fluids into me right away. In came the IV nurse. She might as well have been wearing boxing gloves and a blindfold. That lady couldn't hit a garden hose with a fire axe. After seven or eight tries, I told her she was excused. Actually, I told her to get the hell out of my room and not to ever come back.

One of the regular staff nurses was able, after a little work, to get an IV going in my wrist. I told my nurse that I didn't want her to let that IV technician get within twenty feet of my bed again. I wasn't feeling well and she had just increased my anxiety. Who instructs these people on how to treat people? All they seem to get is mechanical or technical information,

" ... and that, my dear, is the way you find the best vein."

Mom says it's just another case of people not ever having been on the other end of a needle, or bedpan, or scalpel. Detached people, working in the abstract.

Well, listen up medical providers of the world: These are people, real people with feelings and fears and problems you're treating out here. Get some education about being sensitive to people. You might develop some better communications skills while you're at it, too.

Never mind that old, lame excuse about not having enough time. You're just too busy, you say? Remember what the doctor told the nurse when I was four.

"If you don't have time to hold them and comfort them and give them a little love after you've jabbed their butt with a needle, then you don't have time to jab their butt, either."

I wasn't at the hospital when Patsy had Michele admitted, but even before they left, we all knew that there was a definite possibility another surgery was going to be needed to correct the problem.

Since Michele didn't have a fever or any other signs of an illness or infection, we concluded that some mechanical problem was the most likely cause of her distress.

I stayed home, on the phone, because I wasn't about to have a country surgeon — no matter how good he was supposed to be with a knife — open up this very special patient, if I could find a better alternative.

When you're faced with a serious problem to solve, rely on your past successes. Look to your best instincts. What had we done when Michele was threatened twenty years ago? We had gone to the best in the business, Dr. Robert Filler, Michele's surgeon in Boston. But this time, Bob wasn't the first doctor I called.

First of all, Bob is now the Chief of Surgery at The Toronto Hospital for Sick Children, two thousand miles away, and second, Michele was no longer a child. She was a twenty-four year old young adult.

So, instead of calling Bob Filler, I put in a call to the surgeon who had removed my ruptured appendix a few years back and who had, a few years before that, removed Patsy's ailing gall bladder. His name was Dr. George Nardi, a brilliant surgeon who practiced surgery while he trained young surgeons at Massachusetts General Hospital, in Boston.

George Nardi was loved by his patients, respected by his fellow physicians and worshiped by his students. Today, his former students are practicing exceptionally skillful, life saving surgery all around the world.

To this day, I treasure the fact that George Nardi came into our lives. It was an honor for me to have him treat me. And, of course, I'll always be grateful for the special care he gave Patsy, too.

George Nardi was a very special human being, a highly skilled and talented surgeon and a loving, healing physician. The world, and thousands of grateful people are all better because George Nardi decide to become a physician.

But now, in 1989, Michele was the one in trouble so I placed a call to George Nardi's office at Mass General in Boston. I needed a local referral. I knew he'd have a valued former student who would be practicing in Seattle.

The gentle lady who answered the phone told me that she was in the process of closing the office. Doctor Nardi, she told me softly, had given up his practice. He was dying.

I told her to please extend our very warmest regards to the good doctor and to his family. As I remember from the photographs on his desk, George had two sons who were also physicians. I believe he also had a daughter. It may have been his daughter to whom I spoke that day.

The lady on the phone thanked me for calling and for caring. She never said who she was, but there was a sadness in her voice that indicated to me that she was not just losing her employer. When I hung up the phone I cried for a while, just as I'm crying now as I write this part of the story.

That night, after I settled things for Michele, I wrote a personal letter to George Nardi, not even knowing if he would be able to read it. I was sad to hear that the world was losing such a wonderful physician and friend, but it made me feel a little better to tell him what I had in my heart. George Nardi had touched me very deeply. I hope he was able to receive my letter. I never received, nor did I expect, any reply.

A few weeks later I learned that he had died a short while after my call. I hope his passing was as painless and as peaceful as possible. He deserved that, if for nothing else than for all the pain and suffering he had relieved in his practice of medicine. Thanks, George.

After my heartbreaking call to George Nardi's office, I was still faced with my urgent need to obtain a George Nardi clone for Michele. I called Toronto.

Bob Filler came on the line within seconds. He was just as warm, friendly and concerned as if I had seem him the week before. Michele must be one of his personal favorites. The year before, she had sent him an announcement of her college graduation, receiving a wonderful letter of congratulations from him in reply.

"Bob, I'm looking for another Bob Filler or George Nardi or Larry Page. Can you give us a hand?," I asked him after briefing him on her condition and the events which had lead up to her hospitalization.

"It sounds like she needs to be in the hospital, but we've got to get her off the island and out of that local hospital. Those places are great for broken bones and emergency appendectomies, but that's not where a person with Michele's history belongs," he said, without conveying any impression of disrespect for a local, rural hospital. He was just stating a medical fact.

"It so happens that one of my most accomplished students is Chief of Surgery at Childrens Hospital in Seattle," Bob said.

"You know she's not a kid anymore, Bob. She's twenty-four."

There was a pause on the line.

"Really?"

"Really."

"Well, of course it has been that long, hasn't it?

"At any rate," he continued, "he'll know who should see her in Seattle. His name is David Tapper and as soon as we finish talking I'll call him and bring him up to date on Michele's history. Just wait there, I'll have him call you in a few minutes. Let me have your number," he said.

"Remember, Bob, I need the Bob Filler of the northwest."

"We'll do the best we can, Patrick," he said, with a smile in his voice and a touch of embarrassment.

"Sit tight for a few minutes. If I'm unable to reach him right away, I'll call you back. Tell me what they're doing for her at Whidbey General?"

"They've scheduled x-rays and an ultrasound for tomorrow," I told him.

"Those can't hurt. But, if she's going to have any surgery, we're going to get her out of there and into Seattle. I'll call David. Sit tight. And don't forget to let me know how things go with Michele," he said. I was sure happy to have a resource like that at the touch of a telephone.

In a half hour the phone rang. It was David Tapper, M.D., Chief of Surgery, Childrens Hospital, Seattle. He had just spent the last thirty minutes listening to Bob explain about Michele's colorful past. David was as friendly and as open as Bob. It was a joy hearing the concern in his voice. It was as though he had been Michele's doctor for years. In truth, he had trained with Bob after Michele had passed through the system in Boston.

"I'll tell you what I told Bob Filler twenty years ago, David. I don't want a good doctor. I don't want a competent doctor. I want the doctor who operates on your daughter."

"I'll call you back as soon as I can. It may be a hour or so, but I'll get back to you before noon," he said.

"Thanks. You know, you sure remind me a lot of Bob," I told him.

"What the hell," he said, "I should. He trained me." We both laughed.

In about an hour and a half the phone rang. It was David Tapper again.

"I haven't found a guy who has operated on my daughter, but will a guy who's operated on my wife do?" he asked.

"Depends on how you feel about your wife," I said with a smile in my voice.

He laughed.

"We're going to move Michele to The Virginia Mason Hospital in Seattle. I just talked to John Ryan and he's agreed to accept Michele as a patient. He didn't train under Bob at the Brigham, but he did train in Boston, at Mass General. His mentor over there was a fine surgeon. A guy named George Nardi."

"David, George Nardi took out my appendix and my wife's gall bladder. He's one of my heroes. You could not have given me better news."

"Small world, isn't it?" he asked, not expecting an answer.

"What do we do now?" I said.

"John will call you in a few minutes. He's making the arrangements for Michele right now. Keep me informed. Don't forget, I'm here to help, if I can. Remember, I'm out of town until Tuesday, but you're in excellent hands with John Ryan," he assured me.

"I'm sure we are. Thank you very much. Bob was right about you," I told him.

"Thank you. Don't forget to let me know what's happening with Michele. I'm glad I could be here for her."

"Thanks, again, David." We rang off.

When the call from John Ryan came in I heard the same cool sound in his manner that George Nardi had projected at first. It's trained into most of them over at Mass General, I guess.

He said that he wanted to get Michele to Virginia Mason as soon as possible, but he was having a problem finding a room for her.

"We're full," he said. "We haven't one single empty bed in the whole place. I think we're going to have to leave Michele in Whidbey General for the night and then get her in here in the morning. I know there are a couple of people scheduled to go home tomorrow. We may have to go up there and throw someone out," he joked.

"Okay. In the morning it is," I said.

I called Patsy and Michele and told them that we were staying put for the night, but that in the morning we were off to Virginia Mason. I told her of the conversations with Bob and David and John. Pats was very pleased. I didn't have the heart to tell her about George Nardi until that night at dinner. We both cried a little more when I did.

The doctor at Whidbey General who had seen Michele when she checked in had seemed nice enough. He was very open, answering all of our questions with patience, in English. He suspected that what they were going to find was a constriction in the upper portion of her small intestine, brought on by the heavy doses of radiation she had received as a child. It could be, he cautioned, a tumor, an ulcer or something else, unknown, but everything seemed to point toward a radiation induced constriction of the small intestine. If it was a constriction, surgery was indicated.

We should note here that the severe amount of radiation Michele was given as a child to save her life also gave her a severe amount of internal scarring. The problem was probably a large amount of scar tissue which grew, as she continued to grow, and which was now causing a blockage in her intestines, probably somewhere near the opening from her stomach in a section known as the Duodenum.

With Michele's unusual and complex history, the Coupeville doctor agreed that Virginia Mason was a lot better place for her than Whidbey General might be.

The next morning I stayed home to complete arrangements with Virginia Mason. I had several very helpful conversations with two ladies in John's office who were trying very hard to locate an open bed for Michele.

"If you can have her here around noon, I know we'll have space for her. How is she being transported from Whidbey General?" she asked.

"Michele's mom and I will be bringing her in our car," I answered.

"Are you comfortable with that?"

"Of course."

"She has an IV, doesn't she?," she asked.

"Yes. The hospital is putting a heparin block in the IV for the trip. We'll have her there by noon."

"Not before, please. We're playing musical chairs as it is. We need until at least noon," she told me.

"Noon it is and not a minute before. Where do we come when we get to Virginia Mason? And, by the way, how do I get to Virginia Mason?"

She gave me instructions from the I-90 freeway and told me to bring Michele directly to the Admissions Office, someone would be waiting to meet us. I thanked her and called Pats at Whidbey General in Coupeville.

The doctor in Coupeville wrote a very nice note on Michele's discharge papers. He said that Michele was to be transported to Virginia Mason by her parents who are, " ... Confident and capable of doing so." Nice touch, Doc.

When we rolled into the Virginia Mason complex we discovered that Michele had already been admitted by John Ryan's office. Nice service, I thought.

Patsy needed to give the admitting nurse Michele's history and current status so I headed off with Michele to the radiation department on the second floor of the clinic for her Cat Scan.

"We've been waiting for you," the orderly told Michele as we got on the elevator.

The cat scan machine is a marvelous invention. It's a big donut shaped device with a sliding table that goes through the middle of the donut. As the patient passes through the donut, the machine takes a rapid series of x-rays which dissect the body as though you were cutting through a log, removing a small slice. The machine then reproduces that slice on the computer's memory disc as digital information and displays what it sees on a video screen, where it can be enlarged, moved and viewed from several angles.

Instead of using a saw (or a scalpel), they're able to electronically slice a person in half and look at the internal organs on the screen. I found it to be a fascinating procedure.

Michele found the table cold and its unexpected movement, at first, unsettling, but she quickly adjusted. She and her stuffed bear — which had made many trips with her to radiation treatments in Boston — would take several rides through the donut that day.

On the screen, the radiologist and his technician (the technician runs the machine, but isn't allowed to tell you what she sees, that's the doctor's job) showed me what the cat scan (or C-Scan, as they now call it) was seeing inside Michele, electronically.

Besides a small cyst on her right ovary, it saw, in the area where Michele's stomach ended and the small intestine began, that there didn't seemed to be much of an opening at all. It was pinched down to nothing. They also saw, much to my great pleasure and relief, that there was no unusual mass (which is medical lingo for a tumor) in the area. It appeared to be, as the doctor on Whidbey Island had suggested, a radiation-induced constriction of her bowel. Good news, as far as I was concerned.

The day Michele first went to the hospital Patrick had called Reno, where both Teresa and Traci still lived, to tell them what was taking place on Whidbey Island. They, of course, dropped what they were doing and headed immediately for Seattle.

The girls drove straight through the night and arrived the second morning that Michele was in Virginia Mason. Neither one of them is real good at long distance driving, so they were both a little weary when they tumbled into Michele's private room on the twelfth floor after fifteen hours on the road. Michele was very pleased to see them. There is among the three girls, I'm pleased to say, a great deal of love and mutual admiration. It's one of their parents' greatest joys.

Even though the Cat Scan showed exactly what all the doctors thought — and hoped — it would show, they wanted more proof that an operation was absolutely needed before they scheduled surgery. I was happy that they were being so cautious. If we didn't actually want to slice into that battle scarred tummy again, if there was any other way. Our respect for John Ryan's skills was further elevated as we watched him at work.

The plan was to give Michele a day or two to stabilize. Now that she had intravenous fluids running, she wasn't in any danger of dehydrating. The discomfort from the gas was eased by medication. Rushing her off to surgery just wasn't prudent.

That night, Teresa and Traci stayed with Michele until visiting hours were over before coming to the island to get some sleep. When they got to the house they told me about an unpleasant incident with one of Ryan's surgical residents, Adele Douglas, M.D., a woman who was near the end of her training at Virginia Mason. Adele was only days from entering private practice.

To increase the flow of fluids into Michele's system, it was decided to do what's unpleasantly called a cut down. A cut down is a minor surgical procedure where a small incision is made to allow access to a deeper vein than can be found with a needle just below the skin's surface.

A catheter, instead of a needle, is then inserted into the vein and the incision is closed with a suture or two. It's not a very difficult thing to do. But as access to the circulatory system, a cut down lasts longer, which in Michele's case was a big plus, given her weakened veins.

This particular evening, the young Adele Douglas had not wanted an audience while she performed the cut down, insisting that, to keep the area as sterile as possible, Teresa and Traci would have to wait in the hallway, even though Michele wanted her sisters to be there while she underwent this minor surgery. After all, this was a stranger doctor and she was going to do the cut down on the side of Michele's neck.

Michele wanted some family support, but Adele prevailed and all three girls were upset. When they told me about it when they got home that night, I too, was upset with Adele Douglas.

The next morning when I went to the hospital I checked in with Michele and then went off to see if I could have a little chat with our Dr. Douglas. I went first to the nurses station on the twelfth floor.

"Excuse me. Would you please, when you have a moment, page Dr. Douglas and tell her that Michele Nolan's father would like to see her when she has a moment?"

Before the nurse could answer, the young doctor who was standing not far from me at the desk turned and said, "I'm Dr. Douglas. What can I do for you?"

"I'd like a moment of your time to discuss last night, if I may."

"Of course. Go right ahead."

"I think we might want to find a more private place."

"No," she said, being as assertive as possible, "this will be fine."

"Please understand, Dr. Douglas, it's fine with me, but I don't think you want everyone here at the nurses station to hear what I'm going to say to you. But it's completely up to you."

She looked into my eyes for a couple of seconds and then said, "Let's see if we can find an empty room."

We walked down the hallway a few doors and into an unoccupied patient room.

"Now, what's bothering you?" she asked with as much of an air of superiority as she could muster.

"I'd like to explain a few things to you about our family and then talk to you about your actions last night. First, please understand, we are a very close and a very experienced family when it comes to dealing with the medical world."

"Yes," she said, still trying to maintain her attitude of control, "I understand that Michele has had a lot of treatment."

"That's true and I've learned a lot about how to make that treatment the most beneficial for her," I said. "Please don't make the mistake that just because it says M.D. after your name that I'm particularly impressed. If you want our respect you have to earn it and earn it you did not do, last night."

"What happened last night that's bothering you so much, Mr. Nolan?"

"Your insistence that her sisters leave the room while you did the cut down on Michele, for openers."

I was challenging her medical judgment so her defenses came right up, as I knew they probably would. "I wanted to keep the area as sterile as possible. They weren't gowned or masked."

"Neither were you. In fact, you and your little white coat and dress had probably visited several patients with serious infections, bad diseases and you were undoubtedly packing a lot more potential bugs than one might expect to have found on the girls last night. So your little "sterile field" nonsense doesn't hold water, and you know it. You just didn't want them to watch you work."

"They didn't need to be there."

"Yes they did."

"You really think they needed to be there?" she demanded.

"Damn right I do. Let's get one thing very clear here. You are not first in line for consideration. Michele comes first. The family's needs are next and you and the rest of the folks who work here are third."

"I still don't think they needed to be there last night. It's not a very big procedure," she still insisted.

"Michele wanted them to stay with her and that's all that's important to me. If you're uncomfortable having a couple of civilians watch you work, that's your problem, not Michele's," I said.

"Maybe I should speak to Dr. Ryan about it."

"Please, Dr. Douglas, try to understand. I'll see to it that you stay two hundred yards away from Michele at all times if I feel that it would be the best thing for her. I'll fire Ryan, if I feel that's what's necessary, as well. You people have to adjust to us, we will not adjust to you. Our only concern here is for Michele, her well being and her treatment. If you're uneasy having to do a surgical procedure in front of a patient's family, maybe you're in the wrong business. Just remember, your license to practice medicine is going to enable you to make an extremely comfortable living over the next forty or fifty years. If you have to make a few concessions to your patients or to their families from time to time, you're being well paid to make those adjustments."

To her everlasting credit, Adele Douglas looked into my eyes for several seconds while the impact and the full weight of my statements penetrated. She seemed to be giving my position fair consideration.

Without actually backing down she said, "You've given me a great deal to think about. I don't believe I've ever given what you've said much thought before today. Let me have a little while to collect my thoughts on this matter, will you please?"

"Certainly."

"Thank you."

"My pleasure. Have you looked in on Michele yet this morning?," I asked.

"I have her chart right here. I was just headed to her room when you caught me."

I smiled at her, took her arm and said, "Let's go see her together, shall we?"

We walked down the hall toward 1262. Adele asked me a few questions about Michele's childhood surgeries and about the ages of the other girls. Then she asked me what age Traci was when we adopted her.

"Adopted? Do you think one of my kids is adopted?," I teased. "How would you know that?"

My teasing further helped ease the tension which was already quickly dissipating.

You see, Traci and Michael, our two adopted children, are both black. To further confuse people, Traci is married to a wonderful white guy that I think of as a son. When you first encounter the Nolans you can become somewhat confused. We, on the other hand, aren't the least bit confused about it.

As Adele and I walked into her room that morning, Michele was not too happy to see Adele, but she eased up some when I told her about the little chat we had just had.

"I think Dr. Douglas is going to take very good care of you, Michele. We need to set aside what happened last night."

Michele frowned at me.

"It's over, kid. Trust me," I told her.

Adele gave me a quick glance of appreciation. She was learning.

From that day forward, Dr. Adele Douglas was a changed person. She took a special, almost personal interest in Michele. On the very next day, when the IV catheter had not been properly utilized, Adele marched directly down to the nurse's station and demanded to know if anyone knew the cut down had been done in the first place. She was not a happy camper and she let all of them know it. Sometimes a chat with Patrick will have an amazing effect on a person.

The following day they planned to relax Michele into a gentle state of sleep and place a tiny fiber optical tube down into her stomach so they could take a look at the condition of that small intestine and the constriction. They just wanted further proof that all the tests and all the scans and the ultrasound had actually been telling them was the truth.

Teresa and Traci elected to spend the night at the hospital with Michele. Adele had a cot brought up to Michele's room for them. They would take turns sleeping. The girls are very protective of their sister.

Teresa was still upset with Adele Douglas, but I was able to calm her down. I made Teresa agree to give the young doctor another chance before she threw her out the twelfth story window into the street. Charlie, as Patrick calls Teresa, can be one tough customer. I wonder sometimes where she could possible come by that trait.

When we arrived at the hospital the next morning, for what was going to be a tough day, we found Teresa in the waiting area near the elevator. She had been there on the couch since about three that the morning. Traci was sleeping beside Michele's bed on the cot.

"How's Michele?" Patrick asked.

"She's asleep. I was just in there. She's sound asleep, dad. Sitting up."

"Sitting up? In bed?"

"Yup! Sitting up, sound asleep. I never saw anything like it before in my life."

We went down the hall and sure enough, there was Michele, sitting up in bed, not leaning on the pillows nor resting on the raised end of her bed. She was just sitting up in the middle of the bed, fast asleep.

"She's been that way since about two-thirty," Teresa whispered to me.

On the other side of the bed the lump in the covers stirred. In a few seconds the sleepy head of our youngest daughter appeared from the other side of the bed.

"Hi," came Traci's lilting greeting.

"Good morning, honey. How're ya doing?" Patrick asked as he leaned down and gave her a kiss.

"Fine. Michele had a rough night though, but she's been sleeping since about two-thirty — just like that," she laughed as she looked toward her sister. "I don't know how she does that."

Michele looked pretty bizarre, sitting up, sound asleep, without falling over.

Before long Michele opened her eyes. She looked pretty tired.

"Morning," she said softly.

"How are you this fine day?" Patrick asked as he kissed her.

"Sick of all this. Are we going to get the show on the road and get this thing fixed, or what?" she impatiently demanded to know.

"Today's the day, babe," Teresa confidently informed her.

I said, "They're going to put a tiny camera down your throat this morning to see, for sure, what the problem is before they do anything."

"I know what the problem is, mom. I can't eat anything."

More impatience.

"They're just being careful, Michele," Teresa said.

"Well, let's get on with it. I don't think I have any more blood to give these vultures. They were in here twice last night with their little glass vials to be filled. What am I running here, a blood bank for vampires?"

In a few minutes Michele's nurse came in, pleasantly greeting the family, she started to care for Michele.

"Give us a few minutes to get bathed and ready for the day, guys," she said to all of us. Michele's nurse was a very good provider of TLC.

We all kissed Michele as we trouped out to buy the girls breakfast downstairs in the hospital cafeteria. The food at Virginia Mason was — and is — exceptionally good for a hospital. They have a graduate chief running things instead of a sixty year old ex-school cafeteria nutritionist serving up potatoes and chipped beef. It's more like a good restaurant than any hospital cafeteria I've ever seen.

After breakfast Patsy and I met with John Ryan and Adele Douglas to discuss the procedure with the scope that they were going to put down Michele's throat and into her stomach this morning. They just wanted to make sure that surgery was really the only solution.

It's a fairly simple procedure where Michele is only lightly asleep and a thin optical fiber is inserted up her nose and down her throat into her stomach. This was the final test. The final piece of the puzzle to be solved.

A few minutes later we all went to the door of the operating room with Michele, kissed her and wished her luck, then went to the small waiting room just outside the operating suites. John said they'd only be a few minutes. He was true to his word.

When John and the doctor who had actually conducted the examination finished, they gathered the entire family, minus Michele who was still waking up, in a small examining room. John Ryan showed us one of the photographs they had just taken of the constriction, using the fiber optic device.

Next he took out a pen and drew a picture of what they proposed to do, surgically, to correct Michele's problem, which could clearly be seen in the picture.

"We don't want to even attempt to correct or open the constriction. There's just too much risk of damaging a part of this area. It's too fragile, due to all the radiation. If we were to attempt that, it might be too difficult to repair. The tissue around that radiation burn, because that's what it is, a burn, is thin and brittle and not a good candidate for restructuring. We're just going to stay completely away from there. Too dangerous to mess with.

"Instead, if we're all agreed," he said, looking around the room at the whole family, "We propose to take a section of the small intestine that is healthy, somewhere down the line where the radiation did minimal damage, and cut a hole in it so we can attach it to a new opening we'll make in the wall of her stomach. In effect, rerouting the system around the constriction."

John Ryan patiently explained, in detail, what he was going to attempt to do to fix Michele, as he sketched the operation on the back of Michele's chart.

The whole family watched and listened with great attention. Then Teresa asked, "Will that mean that she will have some dietary restrictions or will there be some long term, negative effects on Michele's ability to process the food she eats?"

"Shouldn't be. There may be a short period of adjustment for her digestive system. In other words, we're short circuiting her normal system, bypassing the duodenum, and dumping the digested material from her stomach right into her small intestine. But we believe that should only cause a relatively short period of adjustment for her system."

Young Patrick wanted to know, "Is this a permanent solution or will she have to have another operation in five or ten years?"

"This should solve the problem for the rest of her life. We don't think that there will be any long term side effects nor do we anticipate any reoccurrences of the problem down the line, particularly if we use a portion of the small intestine that hasn't received a major dose of radiation. We're hoping, of course, that we can find some good tissue fairly close to the top. This problem was caused by radiation she received over twenty years ago. That's when the damage was done. But of course, at the time, that radiation also helped saved her life," John reminded us all.

Traci wanted to know, "How long will she have to be in the hospital after this operation?"

"She's in very good health, except for this little blockage, so I would think that she'd be with us ten days to two weeks. Then, after resting well at home, back to better than normal within a month to six weeks."

There were a few other questions about Michele's eating habits — she should stay away from milk products and anything with bubbles for a couple of months we were told.

Then Patsy asked, "When do you propose to do the surgery?"

"Right now. We're all assembled and ready to go. She's already had her pre-op medication with this camera procedure, so, if we're all agreed, we'll just go ahead and do our best to fix Michele."

"We're all agreed. Let us know how it's going, will you?," I said.

"Sure will."

With that, the conference started to break up. Traci went to say what she had to say to Michele, mom went along to tell Michele that she was on her way to surgery, Teresa went to call her husband, Theo and Traci's husband, David to keep them informed.

I walked over to have a private visit with Adele Douglas.

"You're going to be with Michele in surgery aren't you?" I asked, already knowing the answer.

"Absolutely!"

"Then do Michele's father a little favor then, will you, please?"

"Sure."

"Keep an eye on her for me. She's very special."

Adele put her arm around me and gave me a one-armed hug. "I know she is. I'll be right there the whole time. And, please, don't worry, We're going to make sure that's she's just fine."

"I know you will. Thanks for joining the team."

"My pleasure. It's a great team," she said with a genuine warm smile and another one-armed hug to my waist.

I told Michele, who was still very groggy from the effects of the anesthesia they had administered for the scope, that she was headed for surgery. She seemed to know that before I told her.

When we waved goodbye at the entrance to the OR suites, she was looking straight ahead, calm and confident. Traci, of course, was in tears. She's our most fragile team member. I didn't like sending Michele through those doors any more this time than I did the other times. Traci, who had not been there for those first horrible trips through those forbidding doors, hated it.

John had said that he thought the whole procedure would take two hours or so to complete. He also said that it was only a guess, because there was still a lot they didn't know, and wouldn't know, until they actually took a look inside Michele.

We were fairly relaxed, but with an edge of anxiety. Having a great medical team and having been there before helped, but it was still major surgery on a fragile young lady. It would be a tense day for everyone, everyone but Michele that is. She's slept through some of our family's hardest days.

The surgery began around one in the afternoon. We knew we couldn't expect to hear anything before three or three- thirty so we went to lunch — nobody ate very much — and talked about a lot of silly things. Mostly we each just leaned on each other, keeping our own thoughts about what was happening up on the second floor. Then we wondered back to the surgical waiting area on the mezzanine level at Virginia Mason.

Around three-thirty a young woman whom we had never met before appeared in the waiting room.

"You are the Nolans, aren't you? I don't think I can make a mistake about that," she said as she looked around at our family.

"We are the Nolans," Patsy said with a gentle, warm smile as she reached out a hand to touch the young woman's sleeve.

The woman softly mentioned her name, saying that she was an assistant anesthesiologist, part of the team operating on Michele.

"Dr. Ryan wanted me to come out and tell you that everything is going just fine with Michele. It's going a little slower than they thought it might, but it's going just fine. She's doing beautifully. There's no cause for any alarm. It's just going a bit slowly," she said.

How very thoughtful, I thought. This guy Ryan really does understand how our family works. That's nice. Maybe, I thought, sending word out to us had been Adele Douglas' idea. I think it may have been a mutual expression of consideration and thoughtfulness from both of them.

The young lady went on to tell us that Michele was handling the procedure just fine, all signs were very good. She said that she thought the would be finished within another hour or so, but that it might actually be a little longer, but, if it was, not to worry, everything really was going very well. We thanked her and she went back behind the electric doors.

When he had completed his work, leaving Adele and the rest of the team to put the finished touches on the final stitches, John Ryan came out and sat down to tell us what he had done.

"I've never seen such an interesting case. The radiation has completely cooked the right lobe of her liver. It's just shriveled and withered away to almost nothing, but the other lobe has grown and seems to be very healthy.

"We had somewhat of a tough time with the resection because all the tissue in her tummy is quite thin and brittle. That radiation really did a number on her insides. I wanted to be sure that we used a piece of the small intestine that was as unaffected by the radiation as we could find. That took some looking, but we found what we wanted after a while," he calmly said, smiling, as the five of us gathered around him, a few of us sitting on the floor at his feet.

He went on the tell us how brave he thought she was and how lucky we were to still have her and how much he had enjoyed being able to correct the problem. He still wasn't as warm as Larry and Bob — he wasn't ever going to be and we knew that — but he was just what Michele needed this day.

We also knew that he had faced a very difficult surgical situation this day. Only with great skill had he been able to do what most surgeons would not have been able to achieve. This surgery had not been a walk in the park. They had been operating on onion skin and tissue paper. I'm sure Adele Douglas learned a lot on this day from both John Ryan and from

Michele's delicate insides.

In a few minutes, Patsy and I went in to see Michele in recovery, a visit Ryan had arranged. The next few minutes were the only unpleasant ones for us during Michele's stay at Virginia Mason.

While power corrupts, it is said, and absolute power corrupts absolutely, there is another thing about power. Normally when one is given power that person feels the urgent need to exercise it. Such is the case for a lot of people in white uniforms, lab coats and scrub suits. In recovery, we walked right into one such person who thought she needed to exercise a little power.

Patsy and I were unable to find the right recovery room for a minute. The scrub suits who were standing just behind the automatic — Do Not Enter — doors, did not really want to help us, acting somewhat as though they thought we might speak a foreign language. We were, after all, aliens invading their sacred territory. But, with a little persuasion, I was able to get one of the less threatened ones to direct us the the room where our daughter was coming out of the anesthesia. There, beside her bed stood Virginia Mason's "Miss Bitch."

"You'll only be able to stay for a moment!," was her opening line.

It was obvious that while we had Ryan's permission to be there, we sure as hell didn't have this lady's permission. My stomach twisted, but I only asked how Michele's signs were.

"She's doing fine," Miss Bitch forced herself to say.

Pats and I stroked Michele's head, told her we were there, told her she was out of surgery, told her that we loved her, told her she was okay. We were only there to reassure her that her world was whole again, as she came out of her drug-induced sleep.

I kissed her, saying to Pats, "I'll go out and send in Teresa and Traci for a second."

"Absolutely not," said Miss Bitch, who was just waiting for a chance to exercise that power.

"There will be no one else allowed in here and in fact it's time for the two of you to leave."

"Listen to me and listen very carefully, lady," I said very quietly across Michele's bed. "I'm going out and I'm sending in Michele's two sisters for a few minutes so they can see that she's alive. They're going back to Reno in a few minutes and if you think they're leaving without first seeing Michele after this surgery you've got another think coming."

"I'm afraid I won't be able to allow that," she said, failing to get the message.

"I don't give a good God damn whether you want to allow it or not, quite frankly. And if you even open you mouth again I'll have you removed from this position before you can close it, sister. I've been forced to put up with enough people like you in my lifetime. I don't put up with it anymore," I snarled at her softly, pointing my finger directly at her face.

"Would you be happier taking care of your daughter yourself?," she sarcastically threatened.

"If you don't think you can't handle it," Patsy said to her, as coldly as possible, "Maybe we should."

Michele was in an area all by herself. We weren't bothering any other

223

patients and we sure as hell weren't interfering with Miss Bitch's ability to do what she was being paid to do for Michele. Being paid, I might add, by us!

Miss Bitch could see that she was in a fight which she could not win, not without a terrible and very noisy battle, so she backed down.

Without waiting for her to give me permission, I turned and walked out the door and brought Teresa and Traci back to see Michele.

"Dad, what's the matter?" young Patrick asked when I returned to stay with him for the precious few seconds that the girls would be in with Michele.

"Just another obnoxious bitch who doesn't have a clue as to what she's been hired to do."

"Is Michele okay?" he asked, instantly worried that his sister wasn't being given the best of care.

"Shelly's fine. It's just that the nurse who's been assigned to stay with her here in recovery doesn't have a clue about the healing process. She thinks it's all blood pressures and pulse rates. That's why broads like her get stuck in recovery on PMs, where they seldom have to deal with a person who's fully awake," I told him.

"And nobody ever tells them, except, of course, my father," he said with one of his cute little smiles.

In a few minutes, certainly not more than three or four actually, the girls came out, both crying, but relieved that they had seen and talked to Michele before they had to return to Reno.

Next, young Patrick went in for a brief few seconds. He and Michele are very close. They're not just brother and sister, but very, very good friends. In just a minute, Patrick and his mom came back out. We'd see Michele in an hour or so, after she'd been taken back to her room.

We all went downstairs and out of the hospital to have dinner. Teresa and Traci decided to wait until Michele was safely back in her room before they took off for their long drive back home to Reno. I think they secretly just wanted to keep their father out of the hospital, and especially out of the recovery room, until Michele had been moved back up to her room. The girls seemed to eat rather slowly that night.

Michele's system took its own sweet time adjusting to the new plumbing which bypassed the old clog. Each day saw a little progress, but only just a little. Ten days after surgery she insisted on going home to Whidbey Island. She had been sleeping in a hospital bed for almost three weeks and she wanted to get home to her own room and her own water bed.

On the tenth day, they took out the IV, just to see if she was getting enough nourishment by mouth, particularly fluids, to thrive on her own.

She said, "Can I go home now?"

John Ryan and Adele both told her that it might be too soon, but she insisted that she was fine.

"I'll take it easy and I'll eat carefully," she promised them.

I thought it might be rushing things, so did Patrick, but we both knew that Michele can be relentless when she's made up her mind to something.

So, early the next morning, we packed her up and headed for the

Mukilteo ferry and the short ride to Whidbey Island.

I came home from the hospital ten days after the surgery because I was bored silly in that place. Not only was I alone for most of the day, but I wasn't sick anymore. I walked the halls, visited the newborns down in the nursery, went down to the gift shop and waited for my stomach to adjust itself to the new arrangement Dr. Ryan had constructed. I still had an IV in my arm so, each morning, I just took my rolling IV stand in one hand and headed for the elevator. I spent a lot of time looking through the window of the nursery at those cute little newborn babies.

The day they took out the IV I wanted to go home. I went the next morning, but — and I'm a little ashamed to admit it — the doctors were right. My system wasn't ready to be weaned from its bottle of dextrose and vitamins. My stomach just wasn't ready to carry the whole load, at least not just yet.

The second day I was home I tried to eat a regular meal, but it all came back up. The next day my stomach even rejected water. In fact, within two seconds of drinking a glass of water, my stomach sent back a glass of water. Nothing, not even one drop, seemed to stay down. Dad called Dr. Ryan.

I had to spend seven more days in Virginia Mason, as my stomach made the transition to a double-ender. Boy, was that ever a boring week. Boring, that is, except for the last Sunday I was in the hospital.

Dr. Douglas had removed the IV on Friday night since I seemed to be eating just fine now. She said she was sure I was okay, but they wanted to keep me for a few days, just to make sure my stomach wasn't faking it. I agreed not to fuss, if she would let me go home on Monday.

"If you've been able to eat and keep it all down through the weekend, you can get out of here on Monday," she promised with a smile and a soft touch.

I now had a goal.

On Sunday, before noon, my brother Patrick showed up at the door to my room with a brown shopping bag, the kind you get at Nordstrom or some other big department store. He dramatically checked the hall and closed the door, which was a little unusual.

"What do you think you're doing, Safety Pup?" I said, using my favorite pet nickname for him.

"We're busting you out of here, Sis."

"I can't leave until tomorrow," I protested.

"I said, we're out of here. Now."

"Why?" I was grinning. What, I wondered, were they up to now?

"Cause dad and I are here to bust you out," he said very seriously.

"What?" I laughingly asked.

"We're kidnaping you. I brought your clothes. I'll watch the door. You get dressed. Put your robe on over your clothes and keep your slippers on."

"Why?"

I was really giggling now.

"Trust me."

"Right!"

Patrick slipped back out the door and I changed into the loose fitting jeans and shirt he had brought up in the brown bag. I put on my robe and slippers and opened the door a crack. Patrick slipped around the edge of the door, grabbed the empty brown bag, took a note from his pocket which he pinned to my pillow on the empty bed. He then headed me out the door and down the hall toward the elevators.

"Now, pretend we're just going for a visit downstairs to see the new babies," he instructed with great, dramatic seriousness.

"Fine, but where are we really going?" I wanted to know, starting to feel his sense of adventure.

"Shh... Act normal."

Safety Pup really loves this kind of cloak and dagger stuff.

We got in the elevator and when the door closed he said, "Give me that robe and those slippers. Quickly!" He put them into the empty brown bag, handing me my tennis shoes. Then he punched the LOBBY button and the elevator started to descend.

From the lobby, I could see Dad waiting in the front driveway with the car running. When we got in the car, and buckled up, I wanted to know where we were going and what the note said.

"The note's for your nurse. It says if she doesn't call the authorities we'll bring you back for dinner. We're taking you to a movie," my brother told me.

"You're kidding?"

"Not for a second. We thought you deserved a break from that place. We're going to the movies, popcorn and all," Dad said.

I loved the idea. What a great comic adventure. I was spirited out of the hospital like part of a James Bond movie and was being taken to a movie.

"Far out, guys."

When we got back from the theater, four hours later, they hadn't even missed me. They just thought I'd been out wandering around the hospital.

When I told my nurse that I had been to the movies he didn't believe me, at first. Finally I was able to convince him that my brother and father had really smuggled me out so they could take me to the movies. He thought it was a hoot.

The next day, I went home for good. The plumbing was working just fine, thank you. And continues to do so to this day.

Although I don't have the peripheral vision to be a safe driver and I am a little shorter than the average young woman and I have to watch what and when I eat, as I've said all along, it sure beats the alternative.

Epilogue & Reflections

A Father's Perspective:

As a parent, I look back on the last twenty-five years as having been a very special gift. We saw our beautiful little girl dragged to the gates of a terrible inferno, ready to be flung into the fire and lost, when she was only three years old. It was — and I think it always will be to some degree — the most terrifying experience of my life.

Then, less and a year later, we were returned to that abyss of terror, once again by Michele's cancer. We were, with the help of some very special members of the medical world, able to see her snatched again from the flames.

If you're the parent of a child who is seriously ill, I truly hope that we've been able to give you some hope and to bring you some encouragement with Michele's story. That has been our intention.

If you are where we were twenty years ago, stand tough. Desperate battles can be won. Keep your wits about you, trust your instincts and never, never sit passively by and let the medical world behave in a way that you know is not right. Do not let events roll over you. Your child's life may depend on the decisions you make. Be sure they are informed decisions.

Scream and holler, pound on the desk, jump up and down and beat your chest if you must, but take charge, be in control and don't ever be afraid to question, ask or insist on knowing what you need to know.

Above all, never be afraid to say, "Let's get someone else's opinion here."

I would also encourage you to stand by your spouse. It is not the parent's fault when a disease attacks a child. At a time which is extremely difficult for a parent, give the other parent of your child all the support you can. You must be there for each other. It's critical.

There will be times when you can't hold up. At those times, hope that your partner is strong that day. And you must be extra strong on the days when your partner is feeling exhausted. Don't let the illness — or even the loss — of a child tear you apart. Let it bring out your strengths and let it tighten the bond that was there when you brought your child into the world.

If praying helps, pray. But don't put your child's life in the hands of anyone but yourself. That's your job.

Remember, I believe that the strength of will which is most important are the wills of the parents and the patient. If the two of you are strong, it will make your child strong. Stand tough — stand together. These are the times that bond two people together, a lot more then those candlelight dinners on the patio.

Michele didn't die when it looked like there was nothing left for her to do, because we never believed she would die and because she never believed she would die. I believe that. I also believe that she lived because we were able to select the right weapons and the right knights and ladies to accompany her into battle.

The past twenty-five years have been a gift for me.

Michele's life has been a gift for me — and for the world. She's the most tender, sensitive, honest and loyal person I have ever known. In some way, he enriches every life she touches.

Of course, her life has also been a tale of the Perils of Pauline, too. From her walk out into the middle of Lankershim Boulevard when she was two, to the wild, sled ride under the bumper of a speeding car when she was five, to the car crash she survived at eleven to the reconstructive surgery at twenty-five. Coupled with the four major surgeries and the radiation treatments and the chemotherapy, life with Michele, so far, has been a grand, interesting, although sometimes frightening, adventure.

I always wanted to be a parent, from the time I was very young. I love being the father of my wonderful children. It's all I've ever really cared about doing well.

I have known the famous and the humble. I have dined with governors and criminals. I have had a lot of interesting and unusual experiences in my life, but nothing has given me more terror or provided me with more satisfaction than this adventure with Michele.

I love all of my children, each in a very special way. Each one of them is completely different and totally unique. Each of them provide rewards to their father that can not be written about in the English language. Michele, I think it's safe to say is the the most different and the most unique of my children.

Thanks, Michele, for thirty wonderful years.

Now, a special note to you who have read our story.

Thanks for buying this book. A portion of the profits are being donated to the Dana/Farber Cancer Foundation in Boston. If you checked this book out of the library or borrowed it from a friend, send a little something to The Jimmy Fund in Boston for Michele. We've got a lot to repay.

Reflections of a Mother

I remember standing in our front yard on Old Meadow Road on Michele's fourth birthday. Michele was wearing a pretty pink dress.

Lynn Adams, whose children were attending the party, said, "Doesn't she look healthy."

Six months later, the day we brought her home from the hospital after brain surgery, I looked at her and then at the pictures of her we had taken at her birthday party. I couldn't believe it was the same child. Even with the big turban on her head she looked healthy.

It was as though Larry Page had been able to reach in and take each and every cancer cell out of her body.

I remember talking to a woman at Childrens Hospital in Los Angeles whose son was afflicted with a condition that caused his arms and legs to be withered and deformed. I remember how grateful she was that his mind was fine. She had a friend, she said, whose son was retarded. The woman with the retarded son was so happy that her son's body was strong and healthy.

I remember a wonderful gift from Maria Cole. Maria, Nat King Cole's widow, was one of the hosts on Patrick's LA talk show. Maria had arranged to have a huge mechanical dog, that actually walked and sat up, sent to Michele in the hospital. The really wonderful thing about the gift was that Maria had been thoughtful enough to make sure that the store also sent the batteries, too. Batteries, which of course, were sold separately.

Sally Baker, wife of Patrick's old friend and former boss Walt Baker, had her own hit children's television show in L.A. when Michele was ill. Of course, in full costume as the popular character Hobo Kelly, Sally came to visit Michele in the hospital. Before the visit was over, Hobo Kelly visited every kid, on every floor, in every ward at Childrens. She was only with Michele for a few minutes, but she was at Childrens for hours. Thanks, Sal. Your visit gave them all a wonderful lift.

When Michele got all the toys and dolls in Boston, she gave every duplicate to her sister, Teresa, immediately.

In Boston, one of her roommates was a little boy in a respirator — an iron lung. The boy was very sick. Several months later we took a short cut through that part of the hospital and Michele wanted to stop by and see the boy in the iron lung. Of course, the boy was not there.

Michele said, "I wonder where he is. I think he must have gotten all better and gone home."

One day, during the time when Michele was recovering from her brain surgery, Teresa decided that it was time for a family picnic. We packed all the stuff we would need, including a dozen neighborhood kids, and had our picnic in Maida Pringle's lovely garden at the hospital. While Michele's friends weren't allowed to go up stairs, Michele was allowed to come down. It was a wonderful day — both for Michele and for me.

One day I was waiting for Michele just outside of the x-ray department. A father of an ill child was waiting with me.

"Does your daughter have asthma?"

When I told him that she didn't, he said, "You don't know how lucky you are. There is nothing worse than having a child with asthma."

I could have suggested a few things that I thought might qualify as being worse, but I don't think he would have agreed.

One of my most emotional days was the day Michele decided to discontinue the chemotherapy. She said two years was enough, the cancer was gone.

Of course, Dr. Traggis and I had talked about the fact that we were coming to the end of the two year course of treatment. Now, here we were finally at that day.

"So, Dr. Traggis, what do we do now?"

"I don't honestly know. I have never allowed myself to think about getting this far. I'm not sure I ever really thought we would."

With his help, we did.

Thanks, Demetrius. Thanks a million. Thanks for being there for Michele, but thanks, also, for being there for me. I don't think I could have done it without you.

The Reflections of the Patient

Most of what happened to me when I was so young, has faded from my memory, fortunately. The bulk of this story has been told through the eyes of my parents, because a lot of what happened to me affected them so much more deeply then it did me. I was just too young to take it as seriously as I know now it had been.

Oh, I remember a few things. I remember the lights in the operating room. I remember getting all those cards and dolls and toys. I remember a lot of those painful "finger sticks" that were inflicted on my tiny fingers. But I don't remember the terror. I don't remember being terribly frightened or even very scared.

For a long time, when I was young, I didn't want to talk about having had cancer. I was afraid that if I talked about it, it might come back. I know now that I'm an adult, that talking about it will not make it reappear, but when you're a kid, your imagination can work overtime.

I was also fairly certain, as I grew into my teen years, that I would not want to have children. I was concerned that I might pass on the cancer to them. I know now that science says that they think that only the genetic tendency can be inherited.

A year or more before we started to write this book I began to feel that I might be able to help a little child and her family, if they found themselves facing what I faced and what my folks faced, twenty years before. That's the reason mom and dad and I have written this book.

But before we end, let me say this, very strongly. If you have a child who is suffering from a serious illness, whether it's cancer or some other disease, do them the same favor my folks did for me. Tell your child the truth — the whole truth.

If you're real sick, the truth is the most important thing you can have. I'm certain that if I had ever felt that I was being lied to, or was not being told the truth, I would have been scared to death. I might have been frightened or anxious or even terrified. But I wasn't because I knew that my folks were not lying to me. Let me tell you a little story.

When I was twelve, dad wanted to use me in a television commercial. The commercial was being filmed in an attempt to raise funds for research at the The Jimmy Fund. Dad arranged to have several other children, all of whom had been treated or were currently being treated for cancer, appear in the commercial with me.

At the production meeting before we started to film, one of the other kid's mother asked to speak to my dad, privately. Dad took her out into the studio hallway, away from us kids.

"You're not going to use the word, cancer, in this commercial, are you?"

"Yes, we are," Dad told her.

"Well, then, I'm sorry, but my son will not be able to participate."

"And why is that?" asked Dad.

"Because he doesn't know that he has cancer."

Dad was thunder struck.

"But, he's thirteen years old. He goes to The Dana/Farber Cancer

231

Research Institute every week for treatment. His hair is gone. And you think he doesn't know he has cancer?"

"We just can't bring ourselves to tell him that he has it," she said.

"Ma'am, your son knows he has cancer. You're only fooling yourself with this cruel game."

"But he is my son and it's my decision, isn't it?"

"That's true. But as the father of a child who has had cancer, allow me to say just one thing to you."

"What's that?"

"One day, if he doesn't already, your son will deeply resent you for not telling him the truth. Please, please do not continue with this terrible fantasy. Your son is bright and strong and brave. He deserves to know the truth. The truth will make him stronger."

"Maybe when he's older, when it's all over, I may decide to tell him."

"It will be too late by then. It's like waiting until they are in their teens to tell a child that they were adopted. By the time you decide they're old enough to understand, it's too late. By then, the damage is done."

"Well, I'm sorry. I just can't tell my son that he has cancer."

"He knows," Dad gently assured her.

Dad also told her that he was very sorry that her son wasn't going to be able to appear in the commercial.

"He's a great kid. We've all enjoyed meeting him. Good luck."

The lady thanked my dad and took her son home. That woman, just as my dad told her, was making a terrible, irreversible mistake.

It is my fondest wish that the story of a little girl with cancer was able to give you a reason to hope. Thank you for reading my story. If you have a spare dollar or two, please send it along to the wonderful people at:

The Dana/Farber Cancer Institute
44 Binney Street, Boston, MA 02115

Acknowledgements

The Dana/Farber Cancer Research Fund
"The Jimmy Fund"
Boston, MA

Robert Filler, M.D.
Toronto Hospital For Sick Children
Toronto, Ontario, Canada

Larry Page, M.D.
Miami University Hospital
Miami, FL

Demetrius Traggis, M.D.
"The Jimmy Fund"

Norman Jaffe, M.D.
Robert Anderson Hospital — Houston

Robert E. Hittle, M.D.
Childrens Hospital — Los Angeles

John Ryan, M.D.
& his team, including Adele Douglas, M.D.
Virginia Mason Hospital
Seattle, WA

Dr. Alin V. Botoman
Gastroenterology
Virginia Mason Hospital — Seattle, WA

David & Carol Reed

Harvey Kershnar, M.D.

Charlotte Nolan

Lillian Whalen

Charlie Austin

Linda Austin

Pat Meaney

Fran Meaney

Judy Jones

Dr. Seuss

"The Grinch"

"Nani"

Lynn Adams

George & Alma DeGrasse

Gladys of WBZ

Teresa (Nolan) Vancosky

Traci (Nolan) Kelly

Patrick Henry Nolan, VII

Walt & Sally Baker

Maria Cole

Milt Hoffman

Hugh Delregno

Sandra Muir

WBZ-TV & Westinghouse Broadcasting

KHJ-TV
& the gang at "Tempo"
Los Angeles

Childrens Hospital
Boston, MA

Childrens Hospital
Los Angeles, CA

The Nurses & Staff
of Childrens Hospital
Boston - 1969 - 1980

The Nurses & Staff
of Childrens Hospital
Los Angeles - 1969

The "The Jimmy Fund"
Lab Technicians & Nurses
Especially "Pearl"
1969 - 1980

A Kind & Gentle Man in ICU
Childrens Hospital
Los Angeles - 1969

... & all our friends and neighbors who listened, cooked, baked, watched, washed, drove, housed, cared for, cried with, laughed with, cleaned up after and who gave us the support and encouragement that allowed us to help Michele survive her battles with Cancer.

Our Special Thanks To You All!

... we hope you enjoyed the book!

Index:

Photos of Michele, her family & friends....

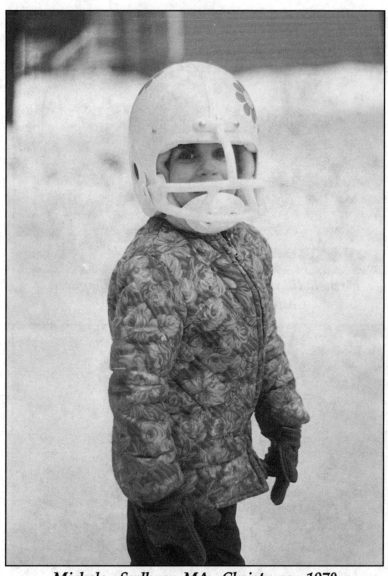

Michele - Sudbury, MA - Christmas - 1970
Ice skating on back yard pond - in flower decked helmet

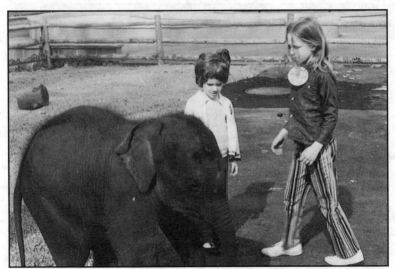

Michele (in wig) & Teresa with Baby Elephant
Children's Zoo - Boston - 1970

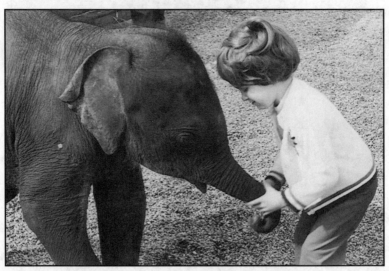

Michele Greeting Baby Elephant
Children's Zoo - Boston - 1970

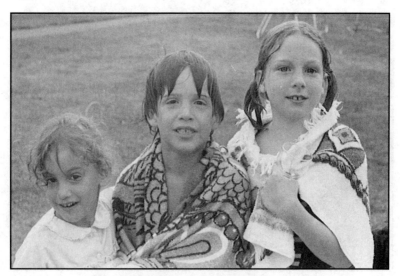

Pam & Mike Adams with Teresa
Sudbury - 1971

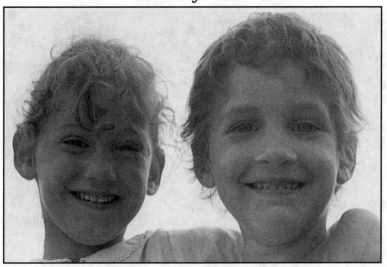

Pam Adams & Michele- 1971

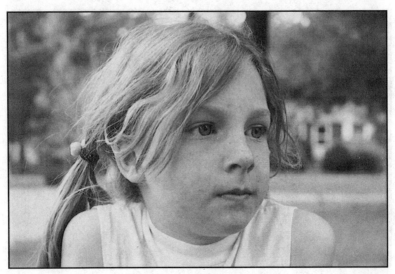

Teresa Nolan - Sudbury - 1972

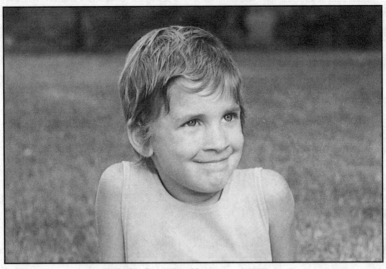

Michele - Sudbury - 1972

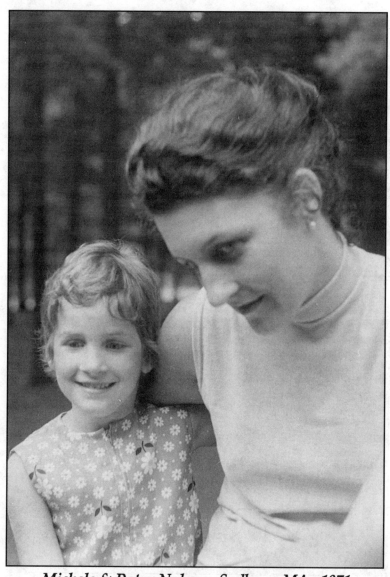

Michele & Patsy Nolan - Sudbury, MA - 1971
Michele's hair has started to return

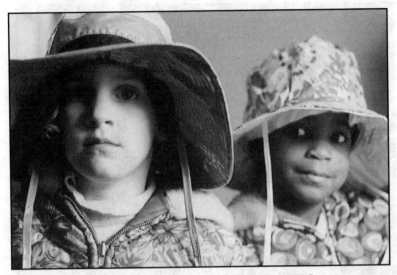

Michele & Traci - Sudbury - 1972

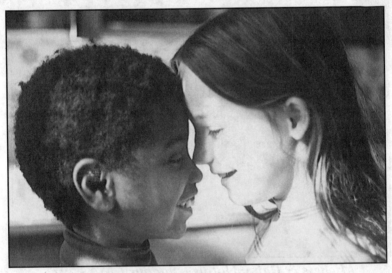

Traci & Jennifer Schultz - Sudbury - 1972

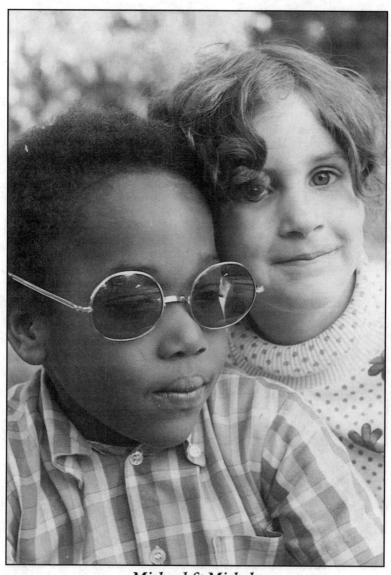

Michael & Michele
Sudbury - 1971

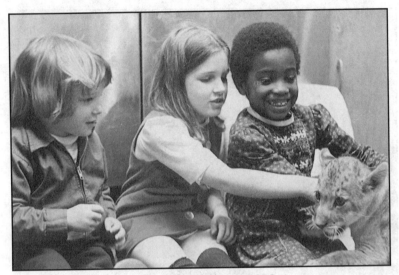

Children's Zoo - 1972
Packet, Michele & Traci with an African Lion

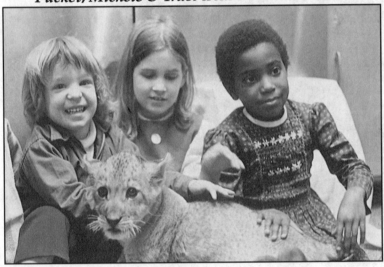

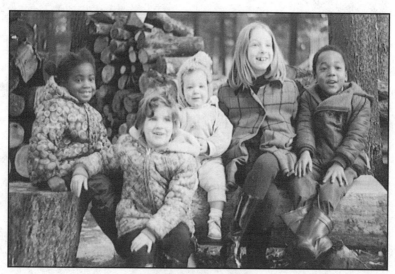

Christmas - 1971
The Five Little Nolans - their first Christmas together

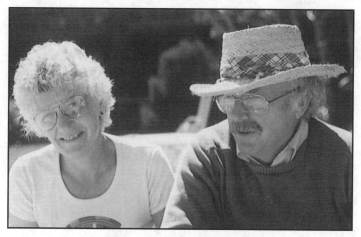

Patsy & Patrick Nolan
Whidbey Island - 1994